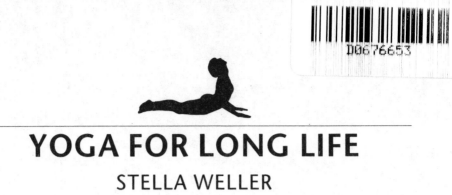

YOGA FOR LONG LIFE

STELLA WELLER

Thorsons

An Imprint of HarperCollins*Publishers*

Thorsons
An Imprint of HarperCollins*Publishers*
77–85 Fulham Palace Road,
Hammersmith, London W6 8JB

Published by Thorsons 1997

1 3 5 7 9 10 8 6 4 2

© Stella Weller 1997

Stella Weller asserts the moral right to
be identified as the author of this work

A catalogue record for this book
is available from the British Library

ISBN 0 7225 3387 X

Printed and bound in Great Britain by Scotprint Ltd, Musselburgh, Edinburgh

CONTENTS

ACKNOWLEDGEMENTS

Many thanks to everyone who helped me with this work. I am particularly grateful to my husband, Walter, to Wanda Whiteley, Jo Kyle, Linda Mellor and the editorial staff at Thorsons; to Jane Bowden and the design team at Thorsons, and to Carol MacFarlane.

LIST OF ILLUSTRATIONS

INTRODUCTION

Older adults represent the fastest-growing segment of the population in many countries today. They are, moreover, living longer than their ancestors did. The number of people in their 70s and 80s has been steadily increasing in industrialized countries, and experts predict that this trend will continue.

The phenomenon is largely due to advances in disease control, better health care and improved nutrition, sanitation and living conditions.

However, some people see life's later years as fraught with loneliness and despair. Contact with children and grandchildren may be limited because of the highly mobile lifestyles of the young. Those who were breadwinners may no longer be needed to provide and may as a consequence feel unwanted. Self-esteem, formerly determined by physical looks and productivity, may start to diminish as the ability to adjust to changes and losses can be seriously challenged and a sense of purposelessness may emerge.

But a growing number of older people refuse to grant permission to society to make them feel unattractive, burdensome and useless. These are the men and women who have decided their own worth and potential. They view life's later decades as a period of integrity, as they reflect on their contributions to family, work force and society. They take pride in their accomplishments and in the wealth of resources (emotional and personal) they have spent many years building up. They are adamant in their refusal to regard this period of life as a time of abandonment and hopelessness. They consider it as offering opportunity for well-earned freedom, continued growth and much-deserved contentment. For them, living longer is not nearly as important as living fully and joyfully.

Life's later years *can* be exciting and infinitely rewarding. But only if you keep fit enough to be able to appreciate them. Few things are, to my mind, sadder than having 'retired' and being financially secure yet not being well enough to profit from the time you finally have at your disposal: not having the capacity to relish your meals, sleep soundly at night or marvel anew at the splendour of a sunset or savour the tranquility of a few moments of solitude at sunrise without equating them with loneliness. How miserable, when time is at last available, not to be able to delight in being able to walk freely and to swing your arms in rhythm or to dance or participate in the many things you had planned.

A growing number of men and women are turning to yoga to help them to acquire and maintain a high level of health, upon which the quality of life undoubtedly depends. They are choosing yoga because it promotes not only physical fitness but mental well-being also.

Yoga is attracting more and more older persons who do not wish to risk injury by practising high-impact (or even 'low-impact') aerobic exercises, but who prefer a kinder, gentler yet effective form of exercise. It is also increasingly appealing to older adults because of its usefulness in the management of pain and other stressors.

More and more, health-promotion programmes are incorporating yoga exercises into their routines for these very reasons. Several of the works consulted during the research for this book suggest the practice of yoga techniques for helping to learn how to relax, to cope with stress and to deal better with anxiety and depression. Many celebrities over fifty attribute their good health, productivity and success partly to their practice of yoga. I see these trends as indicators of the great regard in which yoga continues to be held. Certainly, yoga is ideal for older adults in helping to prevent or to delay the onset of disorders which are considered concomitants of ageing: arthritis, failing vision, depression, high blood-pressure, osteoporosis, and so on. Faithful yoga practice decreases the chance of these and other departures from health being inevitable.

To add a personal note, I can vouch for the beneficial effects of yoga. I am over fifty years of age. I work full-time as a Registered Nurse, doing twelve-hour shifts day and night. In my days off from hospital work, I write books and look after a home and family. I still manage to make and enjoy leisure time. I am seldom ill and I do not take prescription medication. I credit this good fortune in no small measure to the practice of various yoga techniques which I have regularly incorporated into my daily routine for more than twenty years. During difficult times, which are an inescapable part of life, I have found the breathing, relaxation and meditation exercises very useful indeed, helping me to cope effectively while continuing to meet my commitments. Practising the exercises has helped me to retain a sense of self-control, which is a powerful antidote to feelings of being totally at the mercy of outside forces.

The word *yoga* comes from the Sanskrit language. It means 'to integrate'. It is an approach to health care that promotes the harmonious working together of all the body's components. But because it has its roots in the Hindu culture of India, some people believe that it is a religion. This is definitely *not* the case. Yoga is, in fact, non-secretarian and may be practised with full confidence by anyone.

The most popular form of yoga being practised increasingly in the western world in *Hatha Yoga*, or 'the yoga of health'. Its primary goal is to prevent illness, but if illness occurs it helps those who practise it regularly to regain and maintain optimum health. It does this by means of a balanced system of physical and mental training. The 'physical' exercises (*asanas* or postures) benefit not only muscles and joints, but also internal organs, nerves and glands. In addition, they train and discipline the mind so as to improve attention span, concentration and coordination, and they are excellent for preventing a build-up of tension. They are superb for improving posture and carriage. The 'mental' and breathing exercises are perhaps unsurpassed for combating stress, and the relaxation techniques are a useful adjunct to treatments for disorders such as anxiety, depression and hypertension (high blood-pressure).

Because yoga exercises encourage a full focusing on what is being done, they foster a sort of fine tuning-in to yourself. They thus promote a sense of awareness, which alerts you to warning signs of departures from good health. They help you to care for yourself in every aspect of your life. Through regular yoga practice, you acquire a keener sense of wholeness.

Many of the exercises can be incorporated into activities of daily living, to prevent a build-up of tension which often leads to pain. Several of the breathing exercises can be done when driving or waiting (at the doctor's office, or in a queue at the post office, for example), to lessen anxiety, fatigue and frustration. As you become adept at weaving these practices into the fabric of daily life, you will begin to find yoga more and more enjoyable and indispensable. You will feel a new sense of mastery over your life, as you become less dependent on outside agents to keep you healthy and happy, and more and more reliant on your own natural resources: body, mind and breath.

Chapter 8 deals with some disorders that are not uncommon among older adults. The suggestions offered for helping to prevent or to deal with them are intended as a complement to expert medical attention – not as a substitute for it. I encourage you to combine the best that orthodox medicine can offer with yoga and/or other appropriate therapy.

Yoga for Long Life has been written with older adults in mind, but not exclusively for them. It may be used as a practical workbook and handy reference by any one who wishes to practise the exercises in the privacy of his or her own home. It may be utilized as a resource by fitness instructors and health professionals such as doctors, nurses working in general and mental health facilities, and by physiotherapists and community health workers. With modifications, most of the exercises can be practised by people with limited mobility and strength, such as those with arthritis and progressing MS (Multiple Sclerosis), to cite but two examples. *Yoga for Long Life* can, in fact, benefit almost anyone who wishes to recapture and maintain optimum fitness and the joy of living, rather than merely existing and adding years to life.

1

WHY YOGA?

Mature adults who wish to attain and maintain optimum fitness are inclined to avoid forms of exercise that jar their spine and place unnecessary strain on their hip, knee and ankle joints. Now wiser than they were when younger, they are attracted to programmes that take a whole-person approach to well-being, that is, those which involve both body and mind. Wishing to be kinder to their bodies than they perhaps were in their youth, they are consciously choosing gentler yet equally or more effective forms of exercise to help to keep themselves healthy and productive, so that they can live life to the full. This is why, increasingly, older men and women are turning to yoga.

The word 'yoga' comes from the Sanskrit *yuj* which means 'integration' or 'wholeness'. It implies a working together of the mind with all the body's components, and embraces practices that contribute to this harmonious collaboration. In essence, yoga takes a 'whole person' approach, providing those who practise it with the tools to help to maintain a state of balance, or to re-establish it quickly if it is disturbed.

Of the various types of yoga practised in western countries, 'Hatha Yoga' or 'the yoga of health' is the most popular. It consists of 'physical' exercises known as *asanas* or postures, breathing exercises collectively referred to as

pranayama, and various concentration, meditation, visualization and relaxation techniques.

The postures are non-strenuous stretching and strengthening exercises, done in synchronization with regular breathing to provide the working muscles with oxygen. They take each joint through its full range of motion to keep it freely movable. The postures also condition the muscles supporting the joints to keep them firm and strong.

A popular misconception is that because yoga postures are generally slow-moving they do not develop stamina. In fact, it requires more muscular strength to execute a posture slowly than it does to perform it rapidly. As you become more practised and able to 'hold' (maintain) the postures for longer periods, you will find your muscular stamina increasing quickly.

The standing postures (such as the Toe-Finger Posture, Figure 47) and the inverted postures (such as the Half Shoulderstand, Figure 21) are especially useful in this respect. When postures are done in a smoothly-flowing sequence, such as in the Sun Salutations, Figures 36–44, development of cardiovascular stamina is often remarkable and quicker than imagined. (Cardiovascular refers to the heart and blood vessels.)

Each exercise should be done *mindfully*, that is, with full attention given to what is being done. In this way, it is virtually impossible to hurt yourself.

1

The overall immediate effect is to keep not only the muscles and joints of the body's bony framework healthy, but internal structures also: blood vessels, organs, nerves and glands. The cumulative effects include a delay or prevention of the onset of certain disorders associated with ageing, such as arthritis and osteoporosis, and in some cases even a reversal of the condition. Moreover, you work in accord with your own strengths and limitations, aware of being the unique individual that you are. In yoga practice there is no competition.

The breathing, relaxation and meditative exercises enhance the ability to focus, which is imparted by faithful practice of the postures. They are, in addition, superb for diverting your attention from disturbing stimuli and helping you to maintain a sense of self-mastery, particularly in instances where you may start to feel that your body is betraying you. They enable you to conserve energy for constructive use, and to cope effectively with pain and other stressors.

Because yoga has its origins in the Hindu culture of India, many people still harbour the notion that it is a religion. This is not at all the case. Yoga is non-sectarian and may be practised confidently by anyone, no matter what his or her beliefs are. It is, in effect, a science of skilful living. Not surprisingly, therefore, more and more health promotion programmes are utilizing yoga techniques, essentially because they are so conducive to good health and so useful in the effective management of stress. If you are still sceptical, you may wish to consider the fact that thousands of individuals in the western world are practising some form of Japanese martial arts without becoming Buddhists.

Any journey, no matter how long it is, begins from where you now stand. Any stone can eventually be reshaped by a single drop of water dripping steadily on it over time. It is seldom too late to start yoga: even fifteen minutes of faithful daily practice will help to heal and restructure damaged tissues, revitalize mind and body and restore balance and harmony. It will help you to conserve rather than waste your energy, so that you can use it more advantageously. It will provide you with resources for coping well with a variety of stressors and enable you to live to your full potential. Do not, however, expect unrealistically rapid and dramatic results. The benefits you obtain will be proportionate only to the diligence of your practice. Patience and perseverance will bring you rich rewards.

2

PREPARING FOR THE POSTURES

Yoga postures have been practised world-wide for many years. When properly and regularly executed, they bring excellent results. Before attempting to start them, however, please *check with your doctor.*

HYGIENE, SAFETY AND COMFORT

Before starting any exercises, remove any object that might injure you, such as glasses, jewellery or hair ornaments. Wear loose-fitting, comfortable clothing that allows you to move and breathe freely. Whenever possible, practise barefooted.

Empty your bladder and if possible your bowel also. You may take a *warm* bath or shower before exercising, particularly if you feel very stiff. Rinsing or cleansing your mouth and also your nasal passages can be useful before you start.

WHEN TO PRACTISE

Try to practise at about the same time every day (or every other day). Exercising in the morning helps to reduce stiffness which may occur after a night in bed, and will also give you energy for your day's activities. Exercising in the evening induces a healthy tiredness which promotes sound, refreshing sleep. If you find, however, that evening practice is too stimulating, modify your schedule to your greatest advantage: fit the postures in where they seem to work best for you.

Generally, it is best to practise on an empty or near-empty stomach. Before breakfast is a good time, if it suits you. In any case, try not to practise for two or three hours after a meal, depending on its size and content. You may practise about an hour after taking a light snack.

Aim for at least half an hour of practice daily, either in a single session or in two fifteen-minute sessions.

When re-starting after an illness or other interruption, do so very gradually and patiently. Do not try to 'make up for lost time'.

WHERE TO PRACTISE

Choose a quiet place where you can do your exercises uninterrupted for half an hour. The ventilation should be adequate and the lighting soft.

Practise on an even surface covered with a carpet or a non-skid mat. Practise outdoors whenever you can, or on a porch or lawn. From now on, I shall refer to this area as the 'mat'.

HOW TO PRACTISE

One of the things that differentiate yoga postures from most other forms of exercise is the focusing that is required. Multiple repetitions of an exercise, done rapidly while thinking of unrelated activities, are uncharacteristic of yoga.

Begin with a few quiet moments to distance yourself from everyday matters and concerns. Close your eyes, breathe slowly and smoothly and set the mental scene, as it were, for your forthcoming practice. Prior to doing the postures themselves, it is essential to warm up (*see* Chapter 3).

Practise each posture slowly and mindfully, that is, giving full attention to your movements. Synchronize these with regular breathing. When you have completed a posture, maintain it for several seconds to begin with; longer as you become more conditioned. This will be referred to in the exercise instructions as 'hold' the posture.

You should release or come out of the posture equally slowly and attentively, again in synchro-nization with regular breathing. Afterwards, sit or lie down and rest before going on to the next posture. This relaxation period is a significant component of muscle activity, preventing stiff-ness and a build-up of fatigue.

Do not be disheartened if your body does not respond as expected when you first attempt some of the postures. Be patient. The body tends to be forgiving, and persevering with the exercises, *without forcing or straining*, will bring good results in a surprisingly short time.

It is important also to cool down after your exercise session (*see* Chapter 3).

GENERAL CAUTIONS

Always *check with your doctor* before starting yoga or any other exercise programme.

If you suffer from an ear or eye condition (such as a detached retina), you should *omit* the inverted postures such as the Half Shoulderstand (Figure 21) and The Shoulderstand (Figure 33). If you suffer from epilepsy, *omit* rapid breathing as in the Bellows Breath (Chapter 5).

Avoid inverted postures and rapid breathing if you have hypertension (high blood-pressure). If you have heart disease, *avoid* The Bow (Figure 7), The Locust (Figure 25) and the inverted postures.

If you have a hernia, *avoid* The Bow (Figure 7), The Cobra (Figure 10) and The Locust (Figure 25). Also *omit* The Plough (Figure 31) if you suffer from neck pain or have spinal disc problems, and *avoid* The Fish (Figure 17) if you have neck pain or a thyroid gland problem.

Omit the Sun Salutations (Figures 36–44) if you have varicose veins, and if you have venous blood clots *avoid* sitting for any length of time in the folded-legs postures such as the Lotus Postures (Figures 26–28).

If you do suffer from back problems, you might find it helpful to read *The Yoga Back Book* (see the bibliography for details).

Contraindications and cautions for specific exercises are given in Chapter 4.

3

WARMING UP AND COOLING DOWN

Warm-ups are essential preparation for yoga postures. They help to reduce stiffness, increase body temperature slightly and improve circulation. They are therefore useful in preventing the straining of muscles and joints once you begin to practise the postures themselves. They also improve the range of motion of many joints.

Many of the warm-ups which follow can be incorporated into your activities of daily living to prevent a build-up of tension. As such, they can help to prevent the occurrence of many aches and pains which detract from the quality of life. Do all the exercises slowly, smoothly and with awareness, and *do not hold your breath* at any time.

WARM-UPS

SHOULDERS

1 Sit comfortably and hold yourself tall but not stiff. Relax your jaws and hands. Close your eyes or keep them open. Breathe regularly through your nostrils. (You may also practise the shoulder warm-ups while standing).
2 Shrug your shoulders, as if to touch your ears with them. Relax your shoulders.
3 Repeat step 2 at least four times. Rest.

Follow the shrugging exercises with *Shoulder Rotations:*

1 Make slow, smooth circles with your shoulders, in a forwards-to-backwards direction, at least five times. Rest.
2 Make slow, smooth circles with your shoulders, in a backwards-to-forwards direction, at least five times. Rest.

Finish warming up your shoulders with a modified *Horizontal Arm Swing*, as follows:

1 Stretch your arms sideways, at shoulder level.
2 Describe circles in the air, first clockwise then anti-clockwise, five times each. Relax your arms at your sides. Rest.

NECK

1 Sit comfortably and hold yourself tall but not stiff. Relax your jaws, hands and shoulders. Close your eyes or keep them open. Breathe regularly through your nostrils. (You may practise the neck warm-ups while standing).
2 Slowly and smoothly turn your head to your left.
3 Slowly and smoothly turn your head to your right.
4 Repeat steps 2 and 3 at least five times.
5 Look to the front. Rest.

Figure-Eight
Do the Figure-Eight exercise next:

1 Imagine looking at a large figure-eight which is lying on its side in front of you.
2 With your nose, mouth or entire face, trace the outline of the figure-eight in the air, starting with a clockwise motion, at least five times. Rest.
3 Repeat step 2 in the opposite direction, that is, starting with an anti-clockwise motion, at least five times. Rest.

Ear-to-Shoulder
Here is another warm-up to try.

1 Tilt your head sideways, aiming your right ear to your right shoulder. Bring your head upright.
2 Tilt your head sideways, aiming your left ear to your left shoulder. Bring your head upright.
3 Repeat steps 1 and 2 at least five times. Rest.

The Turtle
Finish warming up your neck with this exercise, as follows:

1 Sit or stand tall but not stiff. Relax your shoulders and breathe regularly.
2 Thrust your chin as far forwards as possible, without jerking it. Keep your lips and teeth together without tightening your jaws.
3 Bring your chin back in then tuck it in towards your neck. Do so slowly and smoothly.
4 Go back to your starting position and repeat steps 2 and 3 at least four more times. Rest.

HIPS AND LEGS
The Butterfly
1 Sit on your exercise mat, holding yourself tall but not stiff. Relax your jaws and shoulders. Breathe regularly throughout the exercise.
2 Fold your legs and bring the soles of your feet together. Clasp your hands around your feet; bring your feet comfortably close to your body.

3 Alternately lower and raise your knees, like a butterfly flapping its wings (Figure 1). Do this as many times as you wish, in smooth succession.
4 Carefully unfold your legs and stretch them out. Rest.

Variations
You can also do the *Butterfly* while lying down. Fold your legs and bring the soles of your feet together. Move your knees up and down as many times as you wish (you do not need to hold your feet).

Lying Twist
1 Lie on your back. Stretch your arms sideways at shoulder level. Close your eyes or keep them open. Breathe regularly.
2 Bend your legs. Rest the soles of your feet flat on the mat.
3 Bring your knees towards your chest.
4 Keep your shoulders and arms pressed firmly to the mat as you tilt your knees to one side on an exhalation. Keep your head still or turn it to the side opposite your knees (Figure 2).
5 Inhale and bring your knees to the centre.
6 Exhale and tilt your knees to the other side. Keep your head still or turn it to the side opposite your knees.

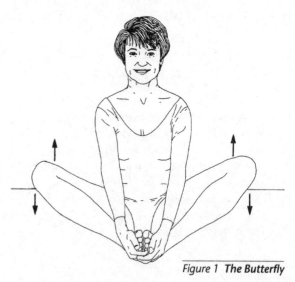

Figure 1 **The Butterfly**

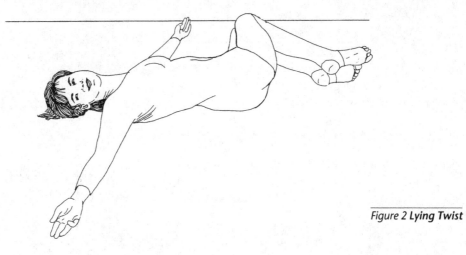

*Figure 2 **Lying Twist***

7 Repeat steps 4 to 6 as many times as you wish, in smooth succession.

8 Stretch out and rest.

Variation I

1 Sit with your legs stretched out in front of you.

2 Bend your legs and lean backwards; support yourself on your elbows.

3 Bring your knees towards your chest.

4 Alternately tilt your knees to left and right, as many times you wish.

5 Stretch out and rest.

Variation II

1 Sit with your legs stretched out in front of you.

2 Bend your knees and rest the soles of your feet flat on the mat, a comfortable distance from your bottom. Rest your hands on the mat to support yourself.

3 Alternately tilt your knees to left and right, as many times as you wish. (Keep your knees together and tilt them as a unit.)

4 Stretch out and rest.

HANDS AND WRISTS
Wrist rotations

1 Sit tall but not stiff. Relax your jaws and shoulders. Close your eyes or keep them open.

Breathe regularly. (You may also practise the hand and wrist exercises while standing.)

2 Rotate your wrists as if drawing imaginary circles with your hands: move your right hand clockwise and your left hand anti-clockwise at least five times. Rest.

3 Repeat the wrist rotations in the opposite direction at least five times: move your right hand anti-clockwise and your left hand clockwise.

The Flower

1 Begin by closing your hands to make tight fists.

2 Slowly with resistance, open your hands like tightly-closed flower buds opening up unwillingly to the rays of the morning sun (Figure 3).

3 Give your palms and fingers a final stretch, and finish by shaking your hands as if expelling dewdrops from them. Rest.

ANKLES

1 Sit tall but not stiff, where you can move your feet freely. Relax your jaws, shoulders and hands. Close your eyes or keep them open. Breathe regularly.

2 Draw imaginary circles with both feet, rotating your right ankle clockwise and your left ankle anti-clockwise at least five times. Rest.

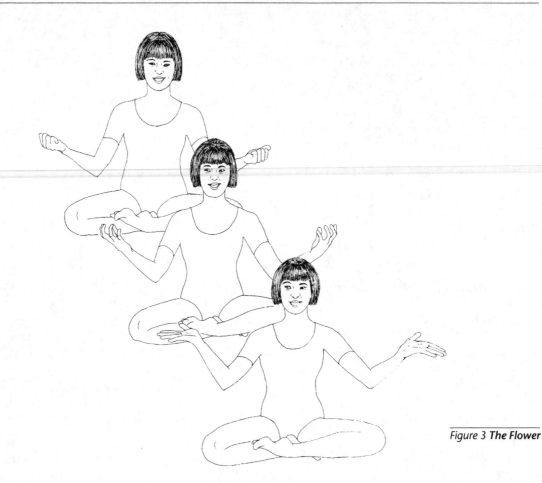

*Figure 3 **The Flower***

3 Repeat step 2 in the opposite direction at least five times: rotate your right ankle anti-clockwise and your left ankle clockwise.

Variation

1 Sit on your exercise mat, with one leg folded inwards. Bend the other leg; pass an arm under the knee and lift the leg off the mat. Rotate the ankle, first clockwise then anti-clockwise, five times in each direction.
2 Repeat step 1 with the other leg and ankle.

WHOLE BODY
Rock-and-Roll

1 Sit on your exercise mat. Breathe regularly. Bend your legs and rest your feet flat on the mat, near your bottom.

2 Pass your arms under your knees and hug your thighs. Tilt your head downwards. Tuck in your chin. Make your back as round as possible.
3 Inhale and kick backwards so that you roll onto your back (Figure 4).
4 Exhale and kick forwards to bring yourself into a sitting position. *Do not land heavily onto your feet* as it will jar your spine. Touch the mat lightly with your toes or feet.
5 Repeat steps 3 and 4 as many times as you wish, in smooth succession. Repeat.

The Fountain

1 Stand tall, with your feet slightly apart and your weight equally distributed between them. Breathe regularly.

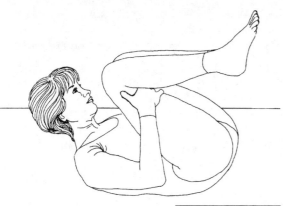

*Figure 4 **Rock-and-Roll***

the other side then forwards, like the flowing water of a fountain (Figure 5). Synchronize the movements with regular breathing.

4 Repeat the rotations anti-clockwise, the same number of times. *Do not* hold your breath.

5 Exhale and lower your arms. Rest.

Also suggested as effective warm-ups are the Sun Salutations (Figures 36–44). Start with two sets and work up to twelve sets.

COOLING DOWN

Cooling down after exercising is very important. It gives the opportunity for static muscle stretching, which enhances flexibility. It allows your heart and blood vessels to return gradually to normal functioning. It helps to prevent problems related to a sudden drop in blood-pressure, such as light-headedness, dizziness or fainting.

Except for the *Rock-and-Roll*, all the exercises given in this chapter can also be used to cool down. Do them slowly, smoothly and with awareness, and in synchronization with regular breathing.

Below are two more cool-down exercises for you to try.

2 Inhaling, raise your arms straight overhead and clasp the fingers of one hand with those of the other.

3 Maintaining the stretch of the arms and body, rotate your upper torso clockwise several times: gently bend to one side, backwards, to

The Stick

1 Lie on your back at full length on your mat. Breathe regularly.

2 Inhaling, sweep your arms overhead and stretch them fully. At the same time, stretch your body to its full length; also stretch your legs and push away with your heels while pointing your toes towards you.

3 Maintain this all-body stretch for several second, but *do not hold your breath*. Keep breathing regularly.

4 Let go of the stretch and resume your starting position, as in step 1 above.

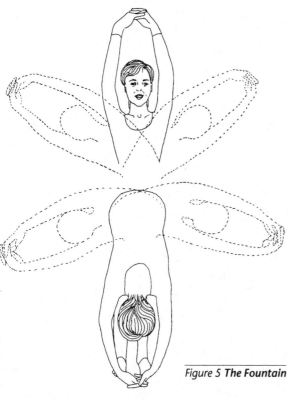

*Figure 5 **The Fountain***

Variation

1 You may do the *Stick* while standing. Stretch your arms overhead; bring your palms together if you can. Stand tall but not rigid.
2 Maintain the top-to-toe stretch for several seconds while breathing regularly.
3 Resume your starting position. Rest.

Rag Doll

Caution You should *omit* this exercise if you suffer from high blood-pressure or if you are prone to dizziness or light-headedness when bending forwards from a standing position.

1 Stand tall. Keep your arms at your sides. Breathe regularly.

2 Tilt your head to bring your chin towards your chest.
3 Let your shoulders droop. Keep your arms and hands limp.
4 Slowly and smoothly curl your body downwards; let the weight of your arms pull you downwards until you are hanging loosely, with your arms dangling.
5 Stay in this posture for several seconds, breathing regularly.
6 Slowly and smoothly uncurl your body, until you are again upright.
7 Sit or lie down and rest.

Finish your exercise session with the *Pose of Tranquillity* (Figure 32).

4

POSTURES

Yoga exercises are called postures or *asanas*, which means 'positions comfortably held'. What differentiates them from some other forms of exercise is that they are done *mindfully*, that is, with full attention given to how they are being done. Because of this, it is virtually impossible to hurt yourself while practising them, since you are alert to the slightest hint of strain. You always work in accord with your limitations.

Also characteristic of yoga postures is the fact that they are done in synchronization with regular breathing. The breath supports the muscular effort and supplies oxygen to the working muscles.

Yoga postures are done slowly and smoothly. You go into a posture or attempt to do so, at which point you stop. You then maintain the posture, for just a few seconds to begin with; longer as you become more practised and comfortable. This phase will be referred to as 'hold' the posture in the exercise instructions.

During the holding period you continue to breathe while maintaining the posture, and you visualize its benefits: the slow, therapeutic stretch of the muscles; the free flow of blood and lymph; the entering of energy and the elimination of waste products through the breath. It is important to create images with which you feel totally comfortable. In time, with faithful practice, you will develop an awareness of beneficial changes in the structures underneath the muscles, such as organs and glands.

When you feel ready to come out of the posture, you do so slowly, smoothly and with awareness, in synchronization with regular breathing.

When first beginning yoga practice, you may find that parts of your body resist your efforts. Try to be patient and sensitive and your body will yield in time. If you attempt to force yourself, or if you become anxious, you will only generate more tension and aggravate the situation. I encourage you to persevere with the exercises, to do the best you can at the moment, and not to be disheartened. Your efforts will bring well-deserved rewards.

For those of you who have not engaged in regular exercise for some time, yoga postures are a marvellously gentle yet very effective way to reverse the effect of disuse atrophy (wasting due to lack of use), stiffening joints, flabby muscles and poor postural habits.

Practising diligently for fifteen to twenty minutes every morning and evening; or half an hour once a day, will help your joints to move freely; increase their range of motion; improve your muscle tone; make you more flexible and reduce aches and pains. Your body will be reorganized and revitalized and will function more economically. Your respiratory (breathing) and nervous systems will be strengthened and you will be able to sleep better. You will be able to deal more effectively and confidently with life's inevitable stressors such as anxiety, frustration and uncertainty. In short, the daily practice of yoga techniques, incorporated into your activities of daily living, will help you not only to add years to your life but also life of *good quality* to your years.

The following postures are arranged in alphabetical order for your convenience. They vary, however, in degrees of simplicity and difficulty. If you have not been exercising regularly for some time, if you are not very flexible, or if you are attempting yoga for the first time, start with the warm-ups (Chapter 3), then try the simpler postures (listed under 'For Beginners' in the suggested Daily Programmes at the end of this chapter). When you become more supple – and you will, in a surprisingly short time, with faithful practice – you may attempt the postures suggested for the Inter-mediate Level, and in time progress to the Advanced Level.

It is very important to remember, at all times, that you are a unique individual with your own strengths and weaknesses, and that the latter can be overcome through patience and practice. Whatever your effort, however small, it is commendable and will pay dividends. Remember *never to strain*. If at first you cannot get into a posture, continue with those with which you are comfortable, and try the difficult posture another time.

Alternate Leg Stretch
What it does
The Alternate Leg Stretch gives natural traction to the spine, which releases pressure on nerves and discs. It therapeutically stretches and tones the back muscles. It also tones and firms the arm and leg muscles and exercises the shoulder and hip joints.

How to do it
1 Sit tall with your legs stretched out in front. Breathe regularly.

2 Fold your right leg inwards and rest the sole of the foot against the left upper thigh.
3 Stretch out your arms and reach for your lower left leg. Exhaling, bend forwards at your hip joints rather than at your waist, and hold on to your outstretched leg. Bend your elbows to help to ease you forwards. Lower your head and relax in the posture (Figure 6).
4 Come out of the posture in reverse, synchro-nizing movement with regular breathing.
5 Stretch out your folded leg and rest.
6 Fold your left leg inwards and repeat the exercise (steps 3 to 5), substituting the word 'left' for 'right' and vice versa in the instructions.

The Bow
Caution You should omit this exercise if you have a serious heart condition or a hernia.

What it does
The Bow strengthens your back and abdominal muscles and keeps your spine flexible. Through gentle yet effective massage, it improves the functioning of organs and glands in the abdomen and small of the back (near the kidneys). It helps to combat constipation, and it expands the chest, thereby facilitating deep breathing, which benefits all body tissues.

How to do it
1 Lie on your abdomen, with your legs comfort-ably separated and your arms alongside your body. Breathe regularly.
2 Bend your knees and bring your feet towards your bottom.

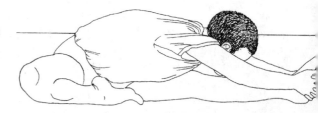

*Figure 6 **Alternate Leg Stretch***

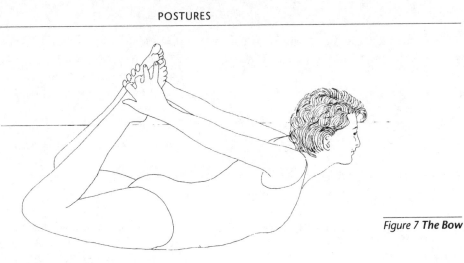

Figure 7 **The Bow**

3 *Carefully* tilt your head backwards. Reach for your feet and grasp your ankles. Keep breathing regularly.
4 *Exhaling*, push your feet upwards and away from you. This action will raise your legs and arch your body (Figure 7).
5 Hold the posture for as long as you are comfortable in it, breathing regularly.
6 Go back to your starting position. Push yourself onto your hands and knees and rest in the *Curling Leaf* posture (Figure 13).

Note This is a challenging posture for intermediate and advanced practitioners. Try it *only* after you have gained some flexibility of your spine. *Do not strain.*

The Bridge
What it does
Excellent for toning the back and abdominal muscles, the Bridge also helps to keep your spine flexible and it gives your body an all-over therapeutic stretch.

How to do it
1 Lie on your back, with your legs stretched out in front of you and your arms relaxed at your sides. Breathe regularly.
2 Bend your legs and rest the soles of your feet flat on the mat, at a comfortable distance from your bottom. Turn your palms down.
3 Inhaling, raise first your hips then *slowly and smoothly* the rest of your back until your torso is fully raised and level. Keep your arms and hands pressed to the mat (Figure 8).
4 Hold the posture for as long as you are comfortable in it. Keep breathing regularly.
5 *Slowly and smoothly* lower your torso, from top to bottom, until it is again flat on the mat. Stretch out your legs. Turn your palms upwards. Rest.

Variation I
Follow steps 1 to 3 of the basic exercise. Once your torso is raised, rest the palms of your hands on your thighs. Straighten your arms. Hold this posture for as long as you are comfortable in it

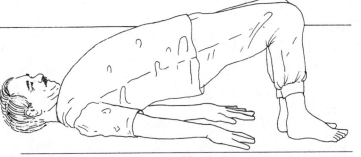

Figure 8 **The Bridge**

and breathe regularly. Slowly return to your starting position (as in step 5 of the basic exercise.)

Variation II
Follow steps 1 to 3 of the basic exercise. Once your torso is raised, stretch your arms straight overhead. Point your knees forward and your fingers backward to give a wonderful stretch to your legs, arms and body. Hold the posture for as long as you are comfortable in it and breathe regularly. Resume your starting position, as in step 5 of the basic exercise.

Chest Expander
What it does
The Chest Expander is wonderful for discouraging a build-up of tension in your upper back and shoulders, and for improving your posture. This exercise is also marvellous for expanding your rib-cage, thereby facilitating deep breathing, with consequent benefit to the respiratory (breathing) and cardiovascular (heart and blood vessels) systems.

The Chest Expander also strengthens the large muscles that enable you to make powerful arm movements when swimming and rowing. These muscles are also involved in vigorous exhalation when singing.

How to do it
1 Stand tall but not stiff, with your feet slightly apart and your weight equally distributed between them. Relax your arms at both sides. Breathe regularly.
2 Inhaling, swing your arms behind you and interlock the fingers of one hand with those of the other.
3 Raise your arms to a comfortable height; resist the urge to bend forwards, but you may bend backwards slightly (Figure 9).
4 Hold the posture for as long as you are comfortable in it, breathing regularly.
5 Relax your arms and body. Rest.

Variations
Unless you suffer from high blood-pressure, or any other condition that prohibits you from hanging your head downwards, you may take this posture a step further and come into a forwards bend while exhaling, keeping your clasped hand and your arms as high up as possible. Breathe regularly while holding the posture for as long as you are comfortable in it. Inhale and return slowly to your starting position.

You may practise the Chest Expander while sitting on a stool, bench, log or other place where you can swing your arms freely behind you. Practise it after you have been engaged in an activity requiring forwards bending, or after sitting at a desk or computer for some time.

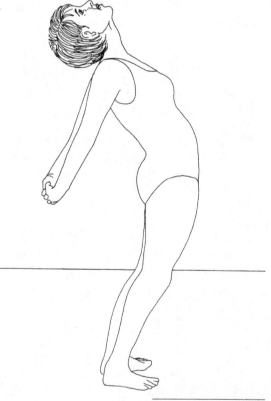

*Figure 9 **Chest Expander***

The Cobra

Caution *Do not* practise the Cobra if you have a hernia of any kind. *Check with your doctor.*

What it does

Excellent for promoting and maintaining flexibility of the spine, the Cobra improves spinal circulation and relieves pressure on nerves and discs. The posture also exercises the shoulder, elbow and wrist joints, thus helping to prevent them from becoming stiff.

Because of the gentle, therapeutic massage it gives your internal organs when the posture is held, the Cobra is also effective in combating constipation.

How to do it

1 Lie on your abdomen. Turn your head to the side. Relax your arms beside you. Breathe regularly.
2 Turn your head to the front and rest your forehead on the mat. Place your palms on the mat, directly beneath your shoulders. Keep your arms close to your sides.
3 Inhaling, *slowly, smoothly and carefully* arch your back: first touch the mat with your nose then your chin as you stretch your neck; then continue the backwards bend until your body forms a graceful arch. *Keep your hips on the mat* (Figure 10).
4 Stay in this posture for as long as you are comfortable in it. Breathe regularly.
5 Come out of the posture in reverse, *slowly, smoothly and carefully*: lower your abdomen, chest, chin, nose and forehead. Turn your head to the side. Relax your arms beside your body. Rest.

Variation

While maintaining the posture during step 4 of the basic exercise, turn your head slowly to the left then to the right, and slowly back to the centre before returning to your starting position.

Notes An excellent position in which to rest following the Cobra is the *Curling Leaf* (Figure 13).

You should try this posture only after you have acquired some flexibility of your spine. *Do not strain.* (Please note that the Cobra is part of the Sun Salutations series, see Figure 42.)

Corrective Prayer Posture

What it does

When you are in this posture your chest is full and round, thus facilitating deep breathing. Your abdomen is at its greatest length, and the pelvic organs are relieved from pressure above.

The Corrective Prayer Posture has the following benefits: it encourages good spinal alignment; it helps to correct postural defects; it promotes muscular coordination and balance and facilitates the distribution of the body's weight along the 132 articulations of the spinal column, thus helping to prevent fatigue. (An articulation is a place of union between two bones.) This posture also gives training in physical and mental steadiness.

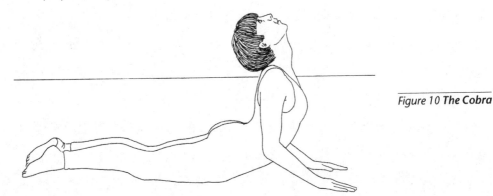

Figure 10 **The Cobra**

How to do it

1 Stand as tall as you can without rising onto your toes. Keep your feet close together and parallel to each other.
2 Check that your head is well poised, i.e. that your chin is neither tucked in nor jutting forwards.
3 Keep your shoulderblades flat.
4 Tilt your pelvis so as to prevent any exaggeration of the spinal curve at the small of your back (lumbar arch).
5 Bring your hands together in front of your breastbone (prayer position). Relax your facial muscles and your jaws, and breathe regularly. Fix your attention on a still object in front of you, or on your breathing, to help to keep you steady (Figure 11).

6 Stay in this posture for about a minute to begin with; longer as you become more comfortable with it. Breathe slowly, smoothly, deeply and quietly.
7 Relax your arms. Rest.

Note You may wish to practise the Stick posture (see Chapter 3) following the Corrective Prayer Posture.

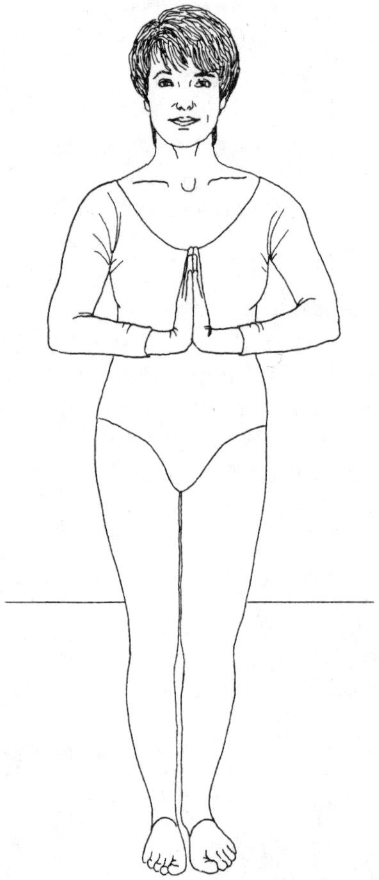

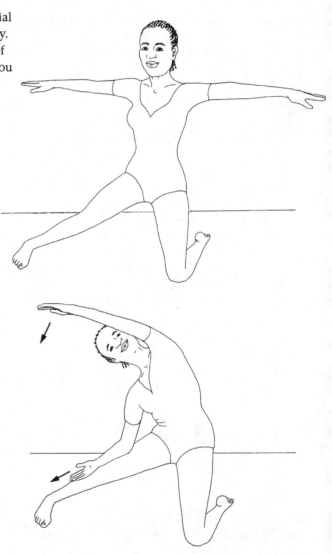

*Figure 11 **Corrective Prayer Posture***

*Figure 12 **Cross Beam***

Cross Beam
What it does
The Cross Beam offers a chance for sideways stretching of the body, thereby contributing to the health of the spine. It conditions the back abdominal muscles and discourages a build-up of fat around the midriff. It also tones and firms the muscles of the arms and legs, and facilitates deep breathing.

How to do it
1 Kneel on your mat. Breathe regularly.
2 Stretch your right leg out to the side; point your toes towards the front rather than sideways, to prevent you from going into a 'split' as you do the posture.
3 Rest your right arm on your outstretched leg; turn your palm upwards.
4 Exhale and bend to the right, aiming your right ear towards your right leg. Raise your left arm and bring it towards your right leg. As you do so, your right arm will slide down the leg. Keep your left shoulder back to ensure a sidewards rather than a forwards bend. Bring the palms together if you can, but *do not strain* (Figure 12).
5 Hold the posture for as long as you are comfortable in it, breathing regularly.
6 Slowly and carefully return to your starting position, as in step 1. Repeat.
7 Repeat steps 2 to 6 on the other side: substitute the word 'left' for 'right' and vice versa in the instructions.

Curling Leaf
What it does
Practised regularly, the Curling Leaf promotes spinal flexibility and good circulation. Through a gentle, therapeutic massage as the posture is maintained, it also helps to combat constipation.

This is an excellent posture in which to rest following backwards-bending postures such as the *Cobra* (Figure 10) and the *Locust* (Figure 25).

How to do it
1 Kneel with your legs together or comfortably apart. Keep your body erect but not rigid. Breathe regularly.
2 Sit on your heels, with your toes pointing backwards (Japanese Sitting Position).
3 Exhaling, lean forwards and rest your forehead on the mat (or turn your head to the side). Relax your arms close beside you, with your palms upturned (Figure 13).
4 Stay in this posture for as long as you are comfortable in it, breathing regularly.
5 Sit up again. Stretch out your legs and rest.

Variation
Follow steps 1 to 3 of the instructions for the basic posture, but modify step 3 so that you stretch your arms straight out in front of you instead of resting them beside you.

Note You may place a cushion, pillow or folded towel or blanket in front of you, on which to rest your forehead or face.

Dancer's Pose
What it does
The Dancer's Pose helps you to develop good concentration and alertness. It also exercises the thigh muscles (quadriceps) which help to straighten the knees.

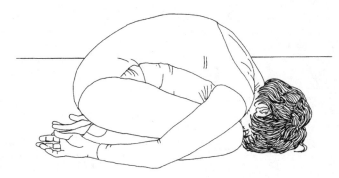

Figure 13 **Curling Leaf**

How to do it

1 Stand tall with your feet slightly apart, and your body weight distributed equally between them. Breathe regularly.
2 Shift your weight onto your right foot. Focus your attention on your breathing to help you to maintain balance.
3 Bend your left leg; hold the foot with your left hand and bring it close to your bottom.
4 Raise your right arm straight upwards (Figure 14).
5 Stay in the posture for as long as you are comfortable in it.
6 Go back to your starting position. Rest.
7 Repeat the exercise, this time standing on your left foot, and raising your left arm. Rest afterwards.

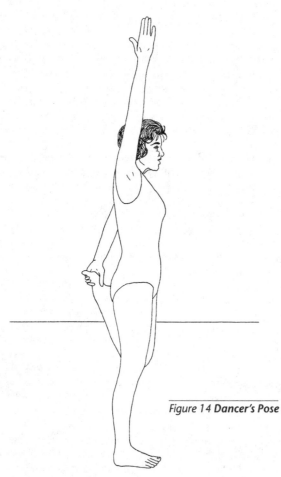

*Figure 14 **Dancer's Pose***

Variation I

In this version of the Dancer's Pose, you *slowly and carefully* bend forwards. Still holding the foot of the bent leg, push it away from your bottom.

Variation II

This easy version of the Dancer's Pose is for those who find it difficult to do balancing postures without the aid of a prop. Hold on with one hand to something stable (such as a post or solid piece of furniture) and use the free hand to grasp your foot, as described in step 3 of the basic exercise.

Variation III

Here is a lying down version of the Dancer's Pose:

1 Lie face downwards and turn your head to the side. You may place a flat cushion or folded towel under your pelvis to reduce the arch of your lower back. Keep your legs close together or comfortably separated. Relax your arms at your sides, or fold them and rest your head on them. Breathe regularly.
2 Bend your legs and bring your heels towards your bottom. As you do so, you should feel a delightful stretch of your thigh muscles.
3 You may alternately bend and straighten your legs, at a slow pace, several times in succession, or you may bend them, hold the position as long as you are comfortable doing so, then rest. Keep breathing regularly throughout the exercise and rest briefly afterwards.

Note When doing balancing postures such as the Dancer's Pose, fix your attention on a stationary object such as a door handle or a picture on a wall, or concentrate on your regular breathing. This will help you to keep steady and maintain your balance.

Dog Stretch

Cautions Omit the Dog Stretch if you suffer from high blood-pressure or have a heart condition, or any disorder that produces light-headedness or dizziness when you hang your head downwards. (Please note that the Dog Stretch is also part of the Sun Salutations, Figures 36–44). *See also* the Half Shoulderstand (page 23) for other cautions related to inverted postures.

What it does

This exercise is wonderful for helping to maintain the elasticity of the hamstring muscles at the back of your legs. When the hamstring shorten, they adversely affect the tilt of your pelvis and may thus contribute to backache.

The Dog Stretch brings a fresh supply of blood to your upper body, thereby benefiting your skin and scalp. It also relaxes tired legs and sometimes can help the entire body.

How to do it

1 Start in an 'all fours' position on your hands and knees. Let your arms slope forwards. Breathe regularly.
2 Tuck your toes in so that they point forwards. Rock backwards slightly. Raise your knees and straighten your legs. Straighten your arms.

Look downwards. You are now in a hips-high, head-low position (Figure 15). Aim your heels towards the mat but *do not strain* the muscles at the back of your legs.

3 Stay in this posture for as long as you are comfortable in it, breathing regularly.
4 Rock forwards gently before returning to your starting position.
5 Sit on your heels, with your toes pointing backwards (Japanese Sitting Position).
6 Rest in the Curling Leaf posture (Figure 13).

The Eagle

What it does

The Eagle gives opportunity to exercise all the joints of your arms and legs to keep them freely movable. Since it is a balancing exercise, it also helps to develop good concentration, nerve-muscle coordination and alertness.

This posture is one of the challenging balancing exercises, and you may wish to try it after mastering the simpler balances such as the Tree (Figure 48).

How to do it

1 Stand tall but not stiff. Relax your arms at your sides. Breathe regularly.
2 Slowly lift your right foot, concentrating keenly in order to keep your balance.

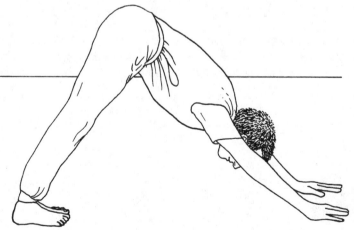

*Figure 15 **Dog Stretch***

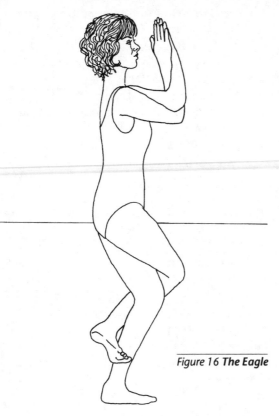

*Figure 16 **The Eagle***

8 Repeat the exercise, this time standing on your right foot and placing your bent right arm inside your bent left arm.

Variation
In this version of the Eagle, you bend forwards *slowly and carefully*. You hold the posture for as long as you are comfortable in it, before resuming your starting position.

The Fish
Cautions *Do not* practise the Fish posture if you have neck pain or an abdominal hernia, or if you suffer from vertigo, dizziness or any balance disorder. *Do not* practise it during the first three days of menstruation. *Check with your doctor* if you have a thyroid gland problem and are considering practising this posture.

What it does
The Fish posture is an excellent exercise for promoting deep breathing and is therefore useful for those who suffer from asthma and other respiratory conditions.

Through a gentle, effective internal massage and stretching of the mid-trunk, the Fish also contributes to the health of organs within your abdomen and pelvis, and combats constipation as well.

The Fish may be a daunting posture if you are coming into yoga for the first time. If you encounter difficulties when attempting this exercise, persevere with simpler back-bending postures such as the Bridge (Figure 8). As your spinal flexibility increases, you will be able to manage the Fish quite easily later. *Do not strain*.

3 Cross your right leg over your left; hook the toes around your left lower leg. Keep breathing regularly and stand as tall as you can.
4 Bend your right arm and hold it in front of you.
5 Bend your left arm and place it inside the bent right arm; rotate your wrists until your palms are together (Figure 16).
6 Hold the posture for as long as you comfortably can, breathing regularly.
7 Slowly unfold your arms then your leg and go back to your starting position. Rest.

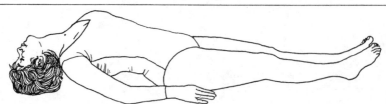

*Figure 17 **The Fish***

How to do it

1 Lie on your back. Stretch your legs out in front. Relax your arms at both sides, with your palms down. Breathe regularly.
2 Bend your arms. Push down on your elbows as you raise your chest and arch your back.
3 *Carefully* slide your head towards your shoulders and feel your neck stretch *gently*. Rest the top of your head on the mat. Adjust your position so that most of your weight is borne by your elbows and bottom, rather than by your head and neck (Figure 17).
4 Stay in this posture for a few seconds to begin with, breathing slowly, smoothly and as deeply as possible. Hold the posture longer when you become more comfortable with it.
5 *Slowly and carefully* return to your starting position.

Note The Knee Press (Figure 24) is a very good position in which to rest and relax after practising the Fish posture.

Variation

Instead of keeping your legs stretched out in front of you, you may practise the Fish in a folded-legs position (*see* the Lotus Postures, Figures 26–28).

Forwards Bend (Sitting)

Cautions Do not practise this posture if you have a hernia or a disorder of the liver, spleen or appendix.

What it does

The Forwards Bend (Sitting) provides gentle traction on the spine, which releases pressure on spinal nerves and discs. It stretches and conditions the back muscles to maintain their effectiveness as spinal supports. In addition, this posture helps to prevent the hamstring muscles (at the back of the legs) from shortening, and is therefore useful in the management of backache (*see* also the Dog Stretch posture, page 19).

The Forwards Bend (Sitting) promotes the health of organs within the pelvis and abdomen.

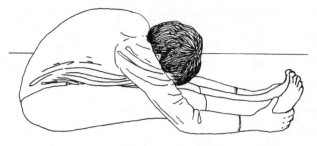

Figure 18 **Forwards Bend (Sitting)**

It helps to keep your hip and shoulder joints flexible; also your elbow joints, if these are bent during the exercise. Ankle joints benefit if you practise the variation in which you hold on to your toes.

Deceptively simple-looking, this posture is best left until you have progressed in your yoga practice. Meanwhile, persevere with easier forwards-bending postures such as the Alternate Leg Stretch (Figure 6) and the Curling Leaf (Figure 13) until your flexibility increases. *Do not strain*.

How to do it

1 Sit tall, with your legs stretched out and together. Breathe regularly.
2 Inhale and raise your arms overhead.
3 Exhale and bend forwards, at your hip joints rather than at your waist, keeping your upper body erect. Reach for your feet.
4 When you can bend no further , hold on to your legs, ankles or feet. Bend your elbows to help to secure your position. Lower your head and relax in the posture, breathing regularly (Figure 18).
5 Stay in this posture for as long as you are comfortable in it.
6 Come out of the posture in reverse, synchro- nizing movement with breathing. Rest.

Variation I

Follow steps 1 to 3 of the basic exercise. Bend your ankles so that your toes point upwards. Hold on to your big toes. Bend your elbows to help you to intensify the forwards bend. Lower your head and maintain the posture while breathing regularly. Come out of the posture in reverse. Rest.

Variation II
After completing your forwards bend, as in step 4 of the basic posture, relax your arms and hands on the mat beside you, rather than holding on to the legs or feet.

Forwards Bend (Standing)

Cautions *Do not* practise this posture during the first three days of menstruation. *Do not* practise it if you suffer from high blood-pressure or any condition that produces light-headedness or dizziness when you bend downwards. *See also* cautions for the Forwards Bend (Sitting).

What it does
The Forwards Bend (Standing) improves the tone of the abdominal and pelvic organs through a two-fold action, namely, increasing intra-abdominal pressure and stretching the back muscles. In addition, it helps to prevent the hamstring muscles (at the back of the legs) from shortening, and is therefore useful in the management of backache (*see* the Dog Stretch posture, page 19). This posture is also of value in weight control and for combating constipation.

This is an advanced posture and so it may prove discouraging to beginners who attempt it. Until you have gained considerable flexibility, continue to practise simpler forwards-bending postures, such as the Alternate Leg Stretch (Figure 6) and the Curling Leaf (Figure 13). *Do not strain.*

How to do it
1 Stand tall but not rigid, with your feet close together and your arms relaxed at your sides. Breathe regularly.
2 Inhale and raise your arms overhead.
3 Exhale and bend forwards, at your hips rather than at your waist (as in the Triangle posture, Figure 50). Do not bend your knees.

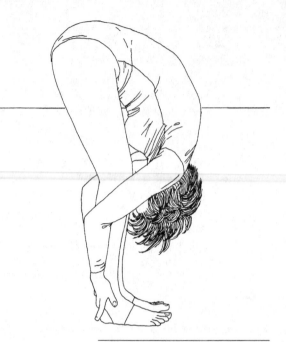

*Figure 19 **Forwards Bend (Standing)***

4 Hold on to your lower legs or ankles. Bend your elbows and gently pull your upper body towards your legs. Avoid exerting too much pressure on your abdomen (Figure 19).
5 Hold the posture for as long as you comfortably can, breathing regularly but not deeply.
6 Come upwards *slowly and carefully* while inhaling. Rest.

Half Moon
What it does
The Half Moon provides a chance to stretch the body sideways, and this is beneficial to both the back and abdominal muscles. It also promotes spinal health, discourages a build-up of fat at the midriff and facilitates deep breathing. In addition, the Half Moon exercises the shoulder joints to help to keep them freely movable.

How to do it
1 Stand tall, with your feet close together and your weight equally distributed between them. Relax your arms at your sides and breathe regularly.

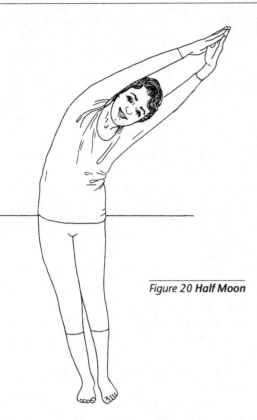

Figure 20 **Half Moon**

What it does

Inverted postures, by summoning the aid of gravitational forces, promote circulation to the upper body and are therefore beneficial to the face and scalp. In the Half Shoulderstand, your back muscles are therapeutically stretched and the muscles of your abdomen and the front of your neck are contracted, thereby revitalizing structures within the trunk and neck. Blood circulation is improved, as well as the functioning of the lymphatic, endocrine and nervous systems.

Some people have claimed that regular practice of this and other inverted postures (such as the Shoulderstand, Figure 33) have helped to restore grey hair to its normal colour.

Note If you are unable or prohibited from doing the Half Shoulderstand for any reason, and wish to try the Dog Stretch (Figure 15) instead, please *check with your doctor* first.

2 Inhale and raise your arms straight overhead. Press your palms together if you can.
3 Exhale and bend sideways, slowly and smoothly, so that your body forms a graceful arch. (Figure 20). Keep your upper shoulder back, and your arm alongside your ear to ensure a sidewards rather than a forwards bend. (Looking towards the upper arm is also helpful.)
4 Hold the posture for as long as you comfortably can, breathing regularly.
5 Return to your starting position. Rest.
6 Repeat steps 2 to 5, bending to the opposite side.

Half Shoulderstand

Cautions *Do not* practise the Half Shoulderstand or other inverted (i.e. hips-high, head-low) postures if you have an ear or eye disorder or if you suffer from heart disease, high blood-pressure or other circulatory disorder. *Check with your doctor.*

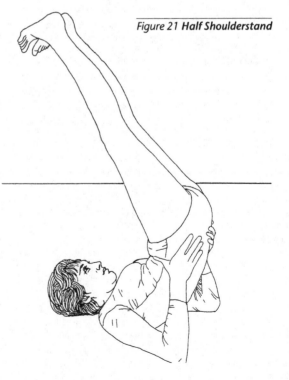

Figure 21 **Half Shoulderstand**

How to do it

1 Lie at full length on your back. Relax your arms at your sides, with your palms turned downwards. Breathe regularly.
2 Bend your knees and rest the soles of your feet on the mat.
3 Bring your knees to your chest.
4 Straighten first one leg then the other so that your feet point upwards.
5 Exhale and kick backwards with both feet at once, until your hips are off the mat. Support your hips with your hand, keeping your thumbs in front (Figure 21).
6 Stay in this posture for as long as you are comfortable in it, breathing regularly.
7 To come out of the posture, rest your arms and hands (palms down) on the mat, close to your body. Keep your head in firm contact with the mat and *slowly and carefully* lower your torso, from top to bottom. Bend your knees and stretch out your legs, one at a time. Rest.

Inclined Plane
What it does
The Inclined Plane gives a wonderful top-to-toe stretch and is excellent for strengthening your arms, legs and torso.

This posture requires strength of the arms, wrists, ankles and legs. If you find it hard or impossible to do at first, persevere with exercises such as the Flower (Figure 3), warm-ups for the hand, wrists and ankles (Chapter 3), and postures such as the Chest Expander (Figure 9)

and the standing balances like the Dancer's Pose (Figure 14) for a period of time until you have acquired the necessary stamina. *Do not strain.*

How to do it

1 Sit tall, with your legs together and stretched out in front. Rest your hands on the mat behind you, with your fingers pointing away from you. Breathe regularly.
2 Press on your palms to help you to raise your body. Hold your hips high. *Carefully* tilt your head back. Your weight should be borne by your palms and feet (or heels), and your body should be level from top to bottom (Figure 22).
3 Hold the posture for as long as you are comfortable in it, breathing regularly.
4 Lower your body to the mat and go back to your starting position. Relax your arms and hands. Rest.

Note *See* the Sun Salutations (Figure 40) for another version of the Inclined Plane.

Knee and Thigh Stretch
What it does
The Knee and Thigh Stretch promotes circulation in the pelvis and abdomen, keeping the bladder, kidneys, prostate gland and other structures in these areas healthy. (Diseases of the urinary system are said to be rare among Indian cobblers who habitually sit in this position.)

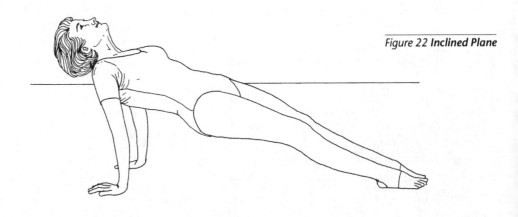

Figure 22 Inclined Plane

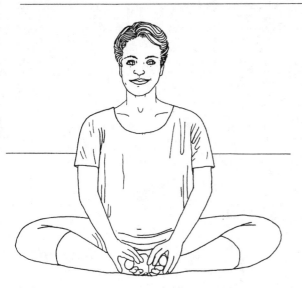

Figure 23 **Knee & Thigh Stretch**

How to do it
1 Sit tall. Stretch your legs out in front of you. Breathe regularly.
2 Fold one leg inwards, placing the heel of the foot as close to your pubic area as you comfortably can.
3 Fold your other leg, bringing the soles of your feet together.
4 Clasp your hands around your feet. Gently pull upwards on your feet as you ease your knees towards the mat (Figure 23). As you do so, you will feel your inner thigh muscles stretch.

5 Hold the posture for as long as you comfortably can, breathing regularly.
6 Ease yourself out of the posture, stretch your legs and rest.

Knee Press
What it does
Superb for relaxing your back muscles, the Knee Press is also effective for helping to rid your body of wind (gas). In addition, it is an excellent counter-posture to do after backwards-bending exercises such as the Cobra (Figure 10) and the Fish (Figure 17).

How to do it
1 Lie on your back, with your legs stretched out in front. Relax your arms at your sides. Breathe regularly.
2 Exhaling, bring first one bent knee and then the other towards the abdomen. Hold your knees or lower legs securely in place (Figure 24).
3 Maintain this posture for as long as you are comfortable in it, breathing gently and regularly.
4 Stretch out one leg at a time and rest.

Variations
Follow steps 1 and 2 of the basic posture. *Carefully* raise your head and bring your forehead towards your knees.
    Hold the posture for as long as you comfortably can, breathing gently and regularly.

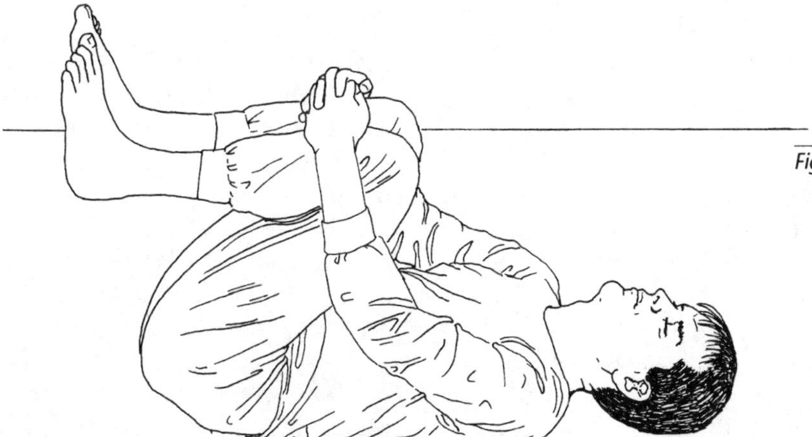

Figure 24 **Knee Press**

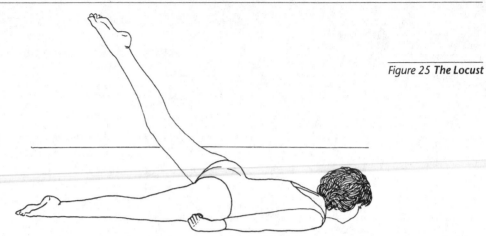

*Figure 25 **The Locust***

Carefully lower your head to the mat, stretch out one leg at a time and rest.

You may also practise the Knee Press with one leg at a time, following the instructions for the basic posture, and also for the variation.

The Locust
Caution *Do not* practise this posture if you have a hernia or a serious heart condition. *Check with your doctor.*

What it does
Wonderful for strengthening your back and legs, the Locust and its variation improve the functioning of internal structures, such as your kidneys, adrenal glands and intestines, and also helps to combat constipation.

How to do it
1 Lie on your abdomen. Turn your head to the side. Relax your arms beside you. Breathe regularly.
2 Turn your head to the front and rest your chin on the mat.
3 Position your arms, kept straight and close together under your body, with your hands made into fists, thumbs down. (Alternatively, rest your arms straight alongside your body, close to it.)
4 Exhale and raise one still-straight leg as high as you comfortably can. Keep your chin, arms, opposite leg and body pressed to the mat (Figure 25).

5 Hold the raised-leg posture for as long as you are comfortable in it, breathing regularly.
6 Lower your leg, relax your arms and hands, turn your head to the side and rest.
7 Repeat steps 2 to 6 with your other leg.

Variation
A more advanced version of this posture requires you to raise both legs together *on an exhalation*.

Hold the posture for as long as you can with absolute comfort, breathing regularly. *Do not strain.*

Return to your starting position, synchronizing movement with breathing. Rest.

Note An excellent posture in which to rest after doing the Locust or its variation is the Curling Leaf (Figure 13).

Lotus Postures
Caution *Omit* these and similar folded-legs postures from your exercise programme if you have venous blood clots.

What they do
The Lotus postures help to tone various nerve centres in your pelvis. By providing a solid triangular base formed by your hips and thighs, with your spine held in good perpendicular alignment, these postures help you to acquire a sense of mind–body balance. They also help you to develop the ability to remain quietly seated

for periods of meditation, and for the breathing exercises.

Because of the firm, stable base which they provide, the Lotus postures encourage good posture and so permit all internal structures to fall into their natural positions and not be cramped. This facilitates circulation and breathing, so that the tissues receive a better oxygen supply. With improved oxygenation, your thinking becomes clearer and your emotions more balanced.

The Perfect Posture

How to do it

1 Sit tall, with your legs stretched out in front. Breathe regularly.
2 Fold your left leg inwards and rest the sole of the foot against your upper right thigh.
3 Fold your right leg inwards and *carefully* place the foot between your left thigh and calf. Rest your hands on your knees or upturned in your lap (Figure 26).
4 Stay in this posture for as long as you are comfortable in it, breathing regularly.
5 Change the position of your legs so that your left leg is uppermost this time.
6 Stretch out your legs and rest.

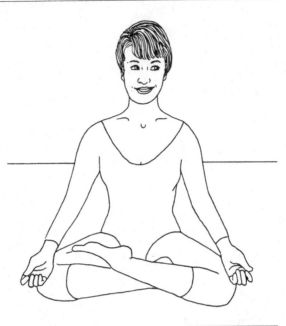

Figure 27 **Half Lotus**

Half Lotus

How to do it

1 Sit tall, with your legs stretched out in front. Breathe regularly.
2 Fold your right leg inwards.
3 Fold your left leg inwards. *Carefully* lift your left foot onto your upper right thigh. Rest your hands on your knees or upturned in your lap (Figure 27).
4 Stay in this posture for as long as you are comfortable in it, breathing regularly.
5 Change the position of your legs so that your right leg is uppermost this time.
6 Stretch out your legs and rest.

Full Lotus

How to do it

1 Sit tall, with your legs stretched out in front. Breathe regularly.
2 Fold one leg inwards. *Carefully* lift the foot onto the upper thigh of the opposite leg.
3 Fold your other leg inwards. *Carefully* lift the foot onto the upper thigh of the opposite leg. Rest your hands on your knees or upturned in your lap (Figure 28).

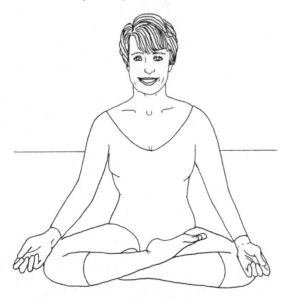

Figure 26 **Lotus (Perfect Posture)**

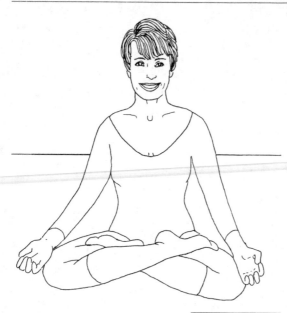

*Figure 28 **Full Lotus***

4 Stay in this posture for as long as you are comfortable in it, breathing regularly.
5 Change the position of your legs.
6 Stretch your legs out and rest.

Notes People who are not accustomed to sitting in folded-legs postures may find that their knees simply will not come close to the floor. They may also find that their back tires easily if they have to sit in these postures for any length of time (such as while doing breathing exercises).

If you are one of these individuals, you will find the following suggestions useful. Place a pillow, cushion or folded towel or blanket on your mat on which to sit. This will help your knees to come close to the floor. If you wish, put a cushion, pillow or folded blanket or towel under each knee for support.

Also, try sitting with your back against a sofa, wall or similar prop until you are able to sit independent of support.

The Mountain
What it does
The Mountain posture tones the pelvic, back and abdominal muscles and discourages fat from building up around the waist and abdomen. It also tones the muscles supporting the internal organs.

In addition, this posture exercises the arm and chest muscles, and facilitates deep breathing by which all the body's cells receive an improved oxygen supply. It also promotes good circulation.

How to do it
1 Sit tall, in any comfortable folded-legs posture, such one of the Lotus postures (Figures 26–28).
2 Inhale and stretch your arms straight overhead, without looking up. Keep your arms close to your ears. Stretch your fingers and bring your palms together if you can (Figure 29).

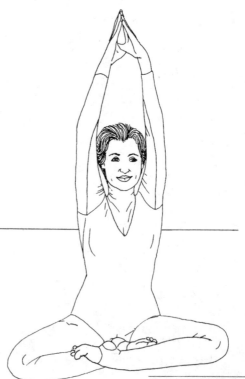

*Figure 29 **The Mountain***

3 Stay in this posture for as long as you are comfortable in it, with your eyes closed or open. Breathe regularly.

4 Lower your arms and relax your hands. Rest.

Variations

You may sit on your heels with your toes pointing backwards (Japanese Sitting Position) to practise the Mountain. You may also practise the posture standing or sitting on a bench or stool, or in the Squatting Posture (Figure 35).

Pelvic Stretch

What it does

The Pelvic Stretch gives a therapeutic stretch to your upper thighs, groins and front of your body. It improves the circulation in the pelvis, thus contributing to the health of the pelvic structures. It also tones and firms the muscles of the back and abdomen.

How to do it

1 Sit on your heels, with your toes pointing backwards (Japanese Sitting Position).

2 Rest your hands on the mat behind your feet, with your fingers pointing away from you. Breathe regularly.

3 Inhale and *carefully* tilt your head slightly backwards. Press on your palms (or fingers)

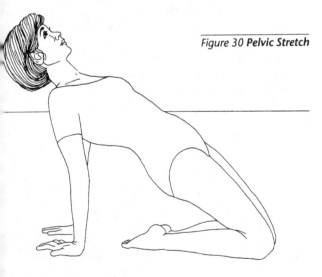

*Figure 30 **Pelvic Stretch***

and raise your bottom off your heels, as high as you can with comfort (Figure 30).

4 Stay in this posture for as long as you comfortably can, breathing regularly.

5 Return to your starting position. Rest in the Curling Leaf posture (Figure 13).

The Plough

Cautions *Do not* practise the Plough if you have a hernia or uterine prolapse, or if you suffer from neck pain or spinal disc problems. *Check with your doctor.*

If you do practise this posture, you should *not* let your hips go beyond your shoulders, as this will place strain on your neck.

What it does

Regular practice of the Plough subjects the spine to a natural, gentle traction which releases pressure on spinal discs and nerves and improves spinal circulation.

The contraction of this abdominal muscles which occurs during the practice of this posture, along with the hips-high, head-low body position, helps to drain and strengthen internal structures and will effectively eliminate wastes. Consequently, the body becomes healthier and the mind clearer.

How to do it

1 Lie on your back, with your legs together and stretched out in front of you. Relax your arms and hands. Turn your palms down. Breathe regularly.

2 Bend your legs and bring your knees to your chest. Straighten your legs so that your feet point upwards.

3 Exhale and kick backwards with both feet at once, until your hips are raised. Keep your arms and hands pressed to the mat.

4 Lower your feet towards the mat behind you. Keep your legs together and as straight as you can without straining (Figure 31).

5 Remain in this posture for as long as you comfortably can, breathing regularly.

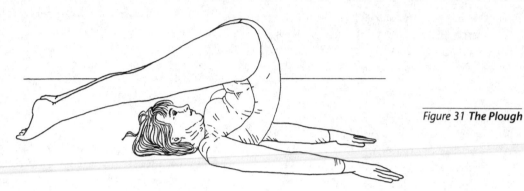

*Figure 31 **The Plough***

6 To return to your starting position, keep your head down on the mat and *slowly, smoothly and carefully* roll your spine onto the mat, from top to bottom. Bend your legs; lower them to the mat, one at a time. Rest.

Note If your toes cannot touch the mat at first, do not be discouraged. They will as your spine becomes more flexible. Meanwhile, try placing some cushions behind you, one on top of the other, so that you can feel your feet touch something. As you make progress, you can remove one cushion at a time. *Do not strain.*

Variation
Instead of keeping your legs together in the completed Plough posture, spread them as wide apart as you comfortably can. Bring them together again when you are ready to come out of the posture.

Pose of Tranquillity
What it does
The Pose of Tranquillity is possibly unequalled as a natural technique for promoting deep relaxation. As such, it is a superb exercise for combating many forms of stress. Practised in the evening, it is excellent for inducing sound, refreshing sleep. It is also very useful in the management of pain and anxiety states, and for counteracting fatigue.

This posture also helps to keep your blood-pressure within normal limits, and is a useful complement to other treatments for heart disorders.

How to do it
1 Lie on your back, with your legs stretched out in front of you and comfortably apart. Relax your arms at your sides, a little way from your body, with your palms upturned. Adjust the position of your head for maximum comfort. Close your eyes. Unclench your teeth to relax your jaws. Breathe slowly and smoothly (Figure 32).

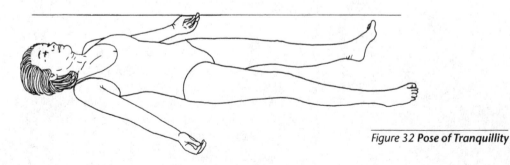

*Figure 32 **Pose of Tranquillity***

This is the basic position. Suggestions for variations are given after the instructions which follow.

2 Push your heels away, bringing your toes towards you. Note the stiffness of your legs and feet as you do so. Maintain this tension for a few seconds. (This step will be referred to as 'hold' from now on.)

3 Let go of the stiffness. Relax your legs, ankles, feet and toes. (This step will be referred to as 'release' from now on.) Let your legs sink with their full weight into the mat.

4 Tighten your buttocks. Hold. Release. Relax your hips.

5 Exhale and press the small of your back (waist) firmly towards or against the mat. Feel your abdominal muscles tighten. Hold as long as your exhalation lasts. Release as you inhale. Relax your abdomen and back.

6 Inhale and squeeze your shoulderblades together. Hold. Release as you exhale.

7 Shrug your shoulders as if to touch your ears with them. Hold. Release. Relax your shoulders.

8 *Carefully* tilt your head backwards. Feel the gentle stretch of your neck. Hold. *Carefully* re-position your head for maximum comfort. Relax your throat.

9 *Carefully* tilt your head forwards, tucking in your chin. Hold. Release. Re-position your head. Relax your neck.

10 Raise your eyebrows to form horizontal wrinkles on your forehead. Hold. Release. Relax your brow. Relax your scalp muscle, which goes from above your eyebrows to the back of your head.

11 Squeeze your eyes shut tightly. Hold. Release. Relax your eyes.

12 Exhaling, open your mouth widely; stick out your tongue as far you comfortably can; open your eyes widely as if staring. Look as fierce as you can. Feel all your facial muscles become tense. (This is the Lion, which may be practised as a separate exercise, in any comfortable sitting or standing position.) Hold the facial tension for as long as your exhalation lasts. Inhaling, pull in your tongue, close your mouth and eyes, and relax your throat and all your facial muscles. Breathe regularly.

13 Stiffen and raise your arms off the mat. Make tight fists. Hold. Release. Relax your arms and hands. Let them sink with their full weight into the mat.

14 Now give your full attention to your breathing. As you inhale slowly, smoothly and deeply but *without strain*, visualize filling your system not only with health-giving oxygen but also with positive forces such as love, hope and joy. As you exhale slowly, smoothly and as thoroughly as you comfortably can, visualize eliminating from your system not only waste products such as carbon dioxide, but also negative forces such as resentment, hopelessness and sadness. Each time you exhale, allow your body to sink a little more deeply into the mat, until every trace of residual tension has vanished.

15 When you feel the need to end your session of deep relaxation, do so *slowly and with awareness*: stretch your limbs in a leisurely fashion and make any other gentle movements you feel the urge to make, such as wiggling your toes and fingers or rolling your head from side to side. When you are ready to sit up, roll onto your side and use your hands to help you. *Do not* come straight up from a supine (lying on your back, face upwards) position, as this may strain your back. Never arise suddenly.

Note and variations

You may practise the Pose of Tranquillity in bed, if you are unwell, or in an easy chair. Modify the exercise instructions accordingly. You may also practise it lying on your back, with your knees bent and your lower legs resting on a padded chair seat or sofa. Use whatever aids and props you need to support your body, particularly your neck and your lower back, so that you feel comfortable. Suitable props include folded or rolled towels, folded blankets, cushions and pillows.

Another good position is to lie on your back, bend your legs, rest the soles of your feet about hips-width-apart, and lean one knee against the other (this relaxes the back muscles). You may also lie on your side, with a pillow between your knees.

Keep a cardigan (or sweater) or blanket and a pair of warm socks nearby. Use them to prevent you from becoming cold as your body cools down during relaxation.

In step 14 of the instructions, use imagery with which you feel most comfortable. You may wish, for example, to visualize yourself lying on a warm, sandy beach in summer, with a soft breeze brushing against your face, hair and body, as you delight in a pleasant memory.

Practise the Pose of Tranquillity any time you need to re-energize yourself, such as after a demanding day or a particularly trying experience that has left you feeling exhausted. Practise it when you feel growing anxiety.

Practise this relaxation technique in a quiet place, where you can be uninterrupted for at least twenty minutes.

When you are well versed in the technique, you may dispense with alternately tightening and relaxing muscle groups, and simply give mental suggestions to the various body parts to let go of tension and relax. For instance, focus your attention on your feet and mentally say, 'Feet, let go of your tightness; relax.' Work from the feet upwards, remembering to include the facial muscles.

You could also record the instructions for the Pose of Tranquillity on a tape-recorder. Speak slowly and soothingly. Listen to the recording as the need arises.

Try this variation called the *Crocodile*.

1 Lie on your abdomen, with your legs fully stretched out and comfortably separated. Place a thin cushion, pillow or folded towel under your hips to prevent an exaggeration of the spinal arch at the small of your back.
2 Fold your arms and rest your head on them. Close your eyes and breathe regularly.

3 Mentally go over your body from feet to head, concentrating on one part at a time, giving each part the silent suggestion to let go of tension and relax completely. Include your feet, legs, hips, upper back, abdomen, chest, arms and hands, neck, scalp and facial muscles.
4 If your thoughts stray, gently guide them back and continue the exercise.
5 Finish with several minutes of slow, rhythmical breathing, letting your body sink more fully into your mat with each exhalation.
6 Roll onto your side and use your hands to help you to get up slowly.

The Shoulderstand

Cautions Refer to the Half Shoulderstand (page 23). In addition, omit this posture if you have an ear problem or suffer from neck pain.

The Shoulderstand is recommended only for those who have been practising yoga for some time, and who have acquired a measure of bodily strength and flexibility. Beginners are advised to persevere with the simpler postures (as suggested in the section entitled 'For Beginners', at the end of this chapter) and to progress to the postures under 'Intermediate Level' (which includes the Half Shoulderstand, Figure 21) before progressing to the full Shoulderstand.

What it does

The benefits of the Shoulderstand (also called the Full Shoulderstand) are the same as for the Half Shoulderstand. In addition, your thyroid gland (located in your neck) receives a gentle, therapeutic massage which enhances its functioning. Since the thyroid gland controls metabolism, all the body's cells and tissues benefit from regular practice of this posture.

How to do it

1 Lie at full length on your back. Relax your arms at your sides, with your palms turned downwards. Breathe regularly.
2 Bend your knees and rest the soles of your feet on the mat.

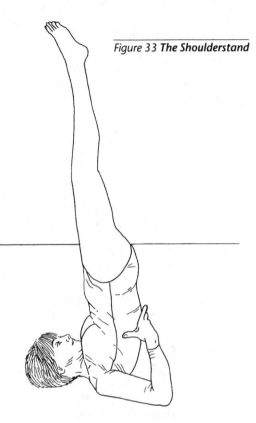

*Figure 33 **The Shoulderstand***

Spinal Twist
What it does
The Spinal Twist (also known as the Twist) is the only yoga posture that requires maximum torsion (twisting) of the spine, first to one side then to the other, thus subjecting the vertebrae (bones forming the spine) to a wide range of motion. This helps to keep the spine flexible and spinal nerves and circulation healthy.

The Spinal Twist also exercises the back muscles and beneficially stimulates the kidneys and the adrenal glands above them. Stimulating these glands results in a sort of 'recharging' of the batteries of the body's cells.

How to do it
1 Sit tall, with your legs stretched out in front of you.
2 Bend your left knee. Rest your left foot on the mat near the outside of your right knee.
3 Exhale and *slowly and smoothly* twist your upper body to the left. Rest both palms on the mat at your left side. Turn your head and look over your left shoulder (Figure 34).
4 Stay in this posture for as long as you comfortably can, breathing regularly.
5 *Slowly and carefully*, untwist to return to your starting position. Rest briefly.
6 Repeat the twist in the opposite direction: follow steps 2 to 5, substituting the word 'right' for 'left' and vice versa in the instructions.

Variations
Instead of resting both hands on the mat, bend one arm and rest the back of the hand against the small of your back (when you twist to the left side, for example, you would bend your left arm). Hold on to the outstretched leg with the free hand.

Instead of keeping one leg outstretched, you can fold it inwards, stepping over it with the opposite foot. For instance, you would fold your right leg when you are twisting to the left. If you wish to modify the position of the hands also, you could rest the back of the left hand against

3 Bring your knees to your chest.
4 Straighten first one leg then the other, so that your feet point upwards.
5 Exhale and kick backwards with both feet at once, until your hips are off the mat. Support your hips with your hands, keeping your thumbs in front.
6 Gradually move your hands, one at a time, towards your upper back, until your body is vertical. Your chin should be in contact with your chest, and your body as relaxed as possible (Figure 33).
7 Hold the posture for as long as you are comfortable in it, breathing regularly.
8 To come out of the posture, tilt your feet backwards. Rest your arms and hands, palms down, on the mat close to your body. Keep your head pressed to the mat. *Slowly and carefully* lower your torso, from top to bottom. Bend your legs and lower them, one at a time, to the mat. Stretch out and rest.

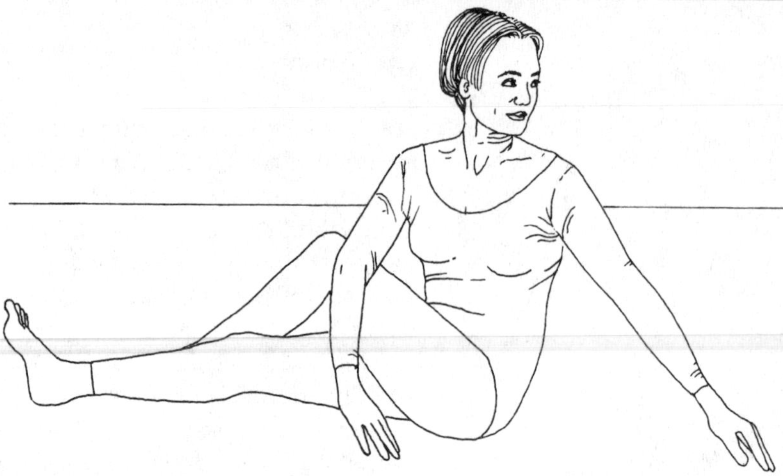

*Figure 34 **Spinal Twist***

the small of your back and hold on to your folded right leg with your other hand (or bring your right arm to the outside of your left leg, bracing it against the leg and holding on to it if possible).

The following is a simplified version of the Spinal Twist but *do not* practise it if you have varicose veins.

1 Sit on your heels with your toes pointing backwards (Japanese Sitting Position). You may place a folded towel or thin cushion between your heels and bottom, and a folded towel under your ankles to take some of the pressure off them.
2 Bring your left hand across the front of your body and tuck the fingers in the cleft formed by your right calf and thigh.
3 Raise your right arm and sweep it backwards, like a swimming stroke. At the same time turn your shoulder, head and eyes to the right to follow the arm movement, as you *carefully* twist your upper body.
4 When you can twist no further, bend your right arm and rest the back of the hand against the small of your back.
5 Stay in this posture for as long as you are comfortable in it, breathing regularly.
6 *Slowly and smoothly* untwist and go back to your starting position.
7 Repeat the twist in the opposite direction: substitute the word 'right' for 'left' and vice versa in the instructions. Rest.

People with varicose veins may welcome the following version of the Spinal Twist:

1 Sit tall on a chair without arms. Face forwards. Rest your feet comfortably on the floor. (If your feet cannot reach the floor, use a folded blanket or cushion on which to rest them.)
2 Exhale and turn your upper body *slowly and smoothly* to the left.
3 When you can turn no further, hold on to the back of the chair with your left hand, and to your left thigh or the side of the chair with your right hand. Look over your left shoulder.
4 Stay in this posture for as long as you are comfortable in it. Breathe regularly.
5 *Slowly and smoothly* untwist and return to your starting position. Rest briefly.
6 Repeat the twist in the opposite direction: substitute the word 'right' for 'left' and vice versa in the instructions. Rest.

Note Here is a tip to help you to remember to which side to twist your body and turn your head: when your left knee is up, twist to the left. When your right knee is up, twist to the right.

Squatting Posture
Cautions *Do not* stay in the Squatting Posture if you have varicose veins. You may, however, practise the variation described after the basic posture. But first *check with your doctor* to make

sure you have no blood clots in your veins. If you do, *omit* this posture and its variation.

What it does
Practised regularly, the Squatting Posture is excellent for keeping your spine flexible and for easing pressure on spinal discs. It is also useful in helping to combat constipation, and it exercises your knee, hip and ankle joints to keep them freely movable.

How to do it
1 Stand with your feet comfortably apart and your weight equally distributed between them. Relax your arms at your sides. Breathe regularly.
2 Inhale and stretch your arms out in front of you, at shoulder level. At the same time, rise onto your toes.
3 Exhale and lower your arms. Lower your body as if to sit on your heels; rest your feet flat on the mat if you can. Arrange your arms for maximum comfort (Figure 35).
4 Stay in this posture for as long as you comfortably can, breathing regularly.
5 Return to your starting position. Sit or lie down and rest.

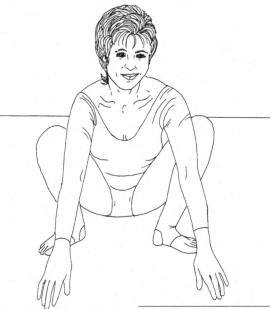

Figure 35 **Squatting Posture**

Variations
Follow steps 1 to 3 of the basic exercise, repeating them several times in smooth succession.

Omit step 4 and finish with step 5.

Notes If you are unsure of maintaining your balance, modify the instructions of the basic exercise and/or its variation by holding on with one hand to a stable prop, such as a solid piece of furniture.

See how many things you can do every day while squatting rather than standing, sitting on a chair or bending forwards. Examples are chatting in the park or on the beach; tidying the lower drawer of a dressing-table or file cabinet; dusting the lower parts of furniture or polishing shoes. I sometimes squat in the bathtub to shampoo my hair with a hand-held shower spray.

Sun Salutations
Cautions *Do not* practise this series of exercises if you have varicose veins, venous blood clots, high blood-pressure or a hernia. *See also* the cautions for the Cobra (page 15) and the Dog Stretch (page 19).

What they do
The Sun Salutations are excellent warm-up and cool-down exercises (*see* page 9). They are splendid for promoting and maintaining flexibility of the whole body and for discouraging a build-up of fat. They are beneficial to the respiratory and circulatory systems, and also to the immune system which protects us from disease. They are, in addition, wonderful for relieving stress.

Practised in the morning, the Sun Salutations help to provide you with energy for the day's activities. Practised in the evening, they promote sound, refreshing sleep.

This series requires a certain degree of strength and flexibility of both the torso and the limbs. Beginners are therefore advised to practise the warm-ups in Chapter 3, and the easier postures (as suggested in the section entitled 'For Beginners' at the end of this chapter) for a period of time before attempting the Sun Salutations. When you do feel ready to try them, start with one or two sets and work up to six or more sets. Remember *not to strain*.

How to do them

1 Stand tall, with your feet fairly close together, and your weight distributed between them. Bring your palms together in front of your chest (Figure 36).
2 Inhaling, raise your arms straight upwards and *carefully* bend backwards to stretch the front of your body; tighten your buttocks to help to protect your back (Figure 37).
3 Exhaling, *carefully* bend forwards and rest your hands on the mat, on the outer side of your feet. Keep your knees as straight as you can, but *do not strain* (Figure 38).

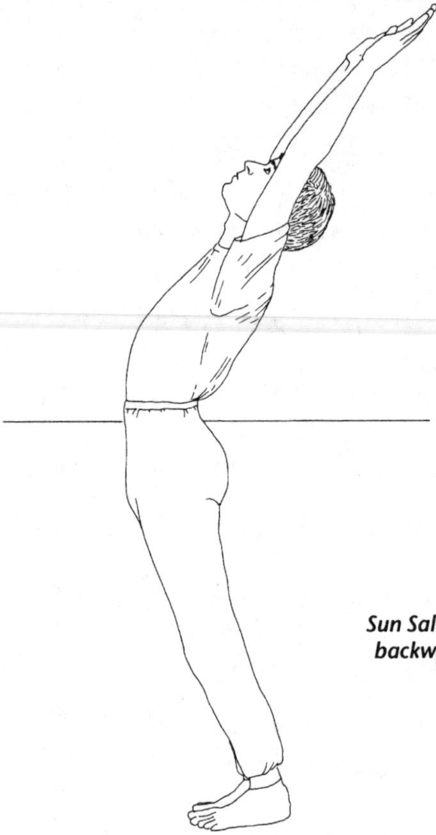

Figure 37
**Sun Salutations –
backwards bend**

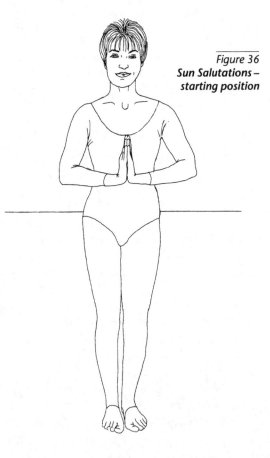

Figure 36
**Sun Salutations –
starting position**

4 Inhale and look upwards. Keep your hands on the mat and step backwards with your left foot; point your toes forwards (Figure 39).
5 Neither inhaling nor exhaling, step backwards with your right foot. Your body should be as level as possible from head to heels (Figure 40).
6 Exhale and lower your knees to the mat. Also lower to the mat your chin or forehead (whichever is the more comfortable), and also your chest. Relax your feet, with your toes pointing backwards (Figure 41).
7 Inhale and lower your body to the mat. *Slowly and carefully* arch your back. Keep your hips and hands on the mat, and your head back (Figure 42). This is the same as the Cobra (Figure 10).
8 Exhale. Point your toes forwards. Push against the mat with your hands to help you to raise your hips. Keep your arms as straight as you

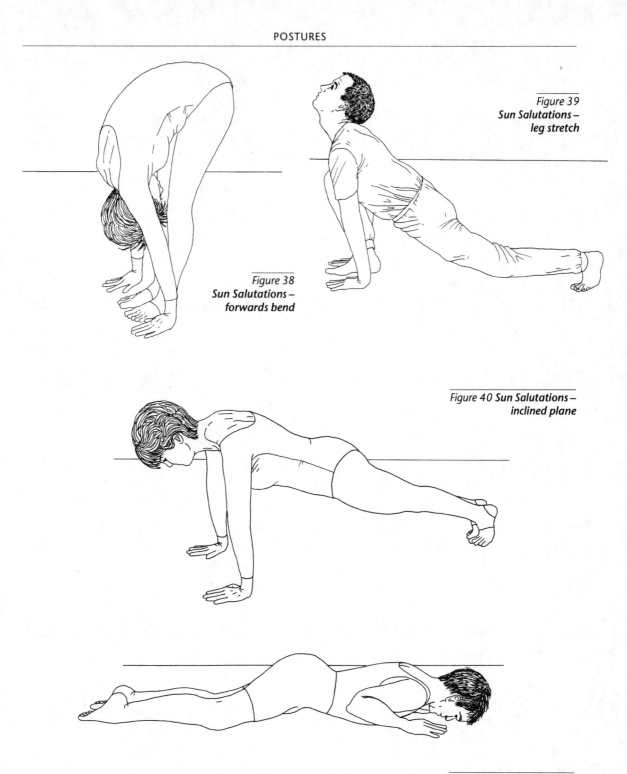

Figure 39
**Sun Salutations –
leg stretch**

Figure 38
**Sun Salutations –
forwards bend**

Figure 40 **Sun Salutations –
inclined plane**

Figure 41 **Sun Salutations –
knee-chest position**

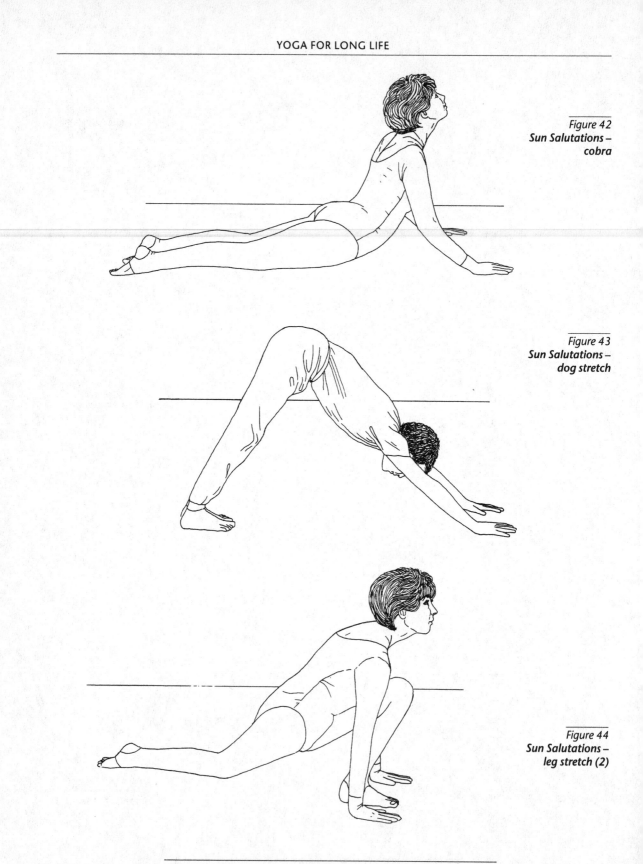

Figure 42
**Sun Salutations –
cobra**

Figure 43
**Sun Salutations –
dog stretch**

Figure 44
**Sun Salutations –
leg stretch (2)**

comfortably can, and your head down. Aim your heels towards the mat, but do not force them down (Figure 43). This is the same as the Dog Stretch posture (Figure 15).

9 Inhale. Look upwards, rock forwards onto your toes and step between your hands with your left foot (i.e. the foot with which you stepped backwards in step 4 of these instructions) (Figure 44).

10 Exhale. Step between your hands with your right foot and come into a forwards-bending position, as in step 3 of these instructions (Figure 38).

11 Inhale. *Carefully* come upwards into a standing position, and move smoothly into a backwards-bending position with your arms raised, as in step 2 of these instructions (Figure 37).

12 Exhale and return to your starting position, as in step 1 of these instructions (Figure 36).

13 Relax your arms. Lie down and rest *or* go on to step 14.

14 Repeat the entire series of exercises one or more times (steps 1 to 13). Rest afterwards.

Notes Read the instructions for the Sun Salutations into a tape recorder, at a slow to moderate pace. Follow the recorded instructions when first trying the exercises, and until you are familiar with them.

When time is limited, you can use the Sun Salutations as the basis for a miniature exercise session. To one or two sets of the series add the Half Shoulderstand (Figure 21) or the Shoulderstand (Figure 33), the Cross Beam (Figure 12) or the Half Moon (Figure 20), the Spinal Twist (Figure 34) and a balancing posture such as the Tree (Figure 48). End with a brief version of the Pose of Tranquility (Figure 32).

You can practise each step of the Sun Salutations as a separate posture: go into the posture, synchronizing the movement with regular breathing; hold the posture for as long as you wish or are comfortable in it; come out of the posture in synchronization with regular breathing and rest briefly before going on to the next posture.

Toe-Finger Posture (Lying)
What it does
The Toe-Finger Posture (Lying) and its variations are excellent for maintaining the tone and elasticity of the hamstring muscles (at the back of the legs), and are therefore beneficial to the health of the back. The posture also keeps the ankle joints strong and freely movable.

The bending of the hips, combined with regular breathing, gives a gentle massage to the abdominal organs, which helps to prevent constipation. The tone of the lower abdominal muscles is also improved, and fat build-up is discouraged.

You may find this posture difficult to do if you have tight hamstring muscles (at the back of your legs). Until your hamstrings lengthen, faithful practice of the ankle warm-ups (Chapter 3) and postures such as the Alternate Leg Stretch (Figure 6) and the Dog Stretch (Figure 15) will condition your legs in preparation for all the Toe-Finger postures (Figures 45, 46 and 47). Keep trying, but *do not strain*.

How to do it
1 Lie on your back, with your legs stretched out in front of you and your arms relaxed at your sides. Breathe regularly.

2 Bend your legs and rest the soles of your feet flat on the mat.

3 Bring first one knee then the other towards your chest.

4 Tuck the fingers of your left hand under the toes of your left foot; do the same with your right fingers and toes.

5 Holding your toes securely, *slowly and carefully* straighten your legs (Figure 45). *Do not strain*. You will be able to straighten your legs fully as you become more flexible with regular practice.

6 Hold the posture for as long as you are comfortable in it, breathing regularly.

7 Release the hold on your toes, bend your legs and rest the soles of your feet on the mat, one at a time.

8 Stretch out your legs and rest.

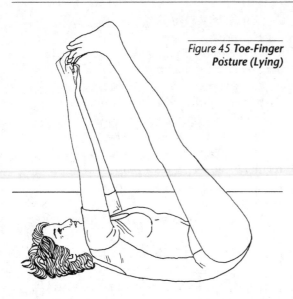

Figure 45 **Toe-Finger Posture (Lying)**

How to do it

1 Sit with your legs bent and the soles of your feet flat on the mat. Breathe regularly.
2 Bring your knees towards your chest. At the same time, tilt backwards a little so that your feet lift off the mat and you are balancing on your bottom.
3 Tuck the fingers of your left hand under your left toes; do the same with your right fingers and toes.
4 Holding your toes securely, *slowly and carefully* straighten your legs (Figure 46).
5 Hold the posture for as long as you comfortably can, breathing regularly.
6 Release the hold on your toes, bring your knees to your chest and resume your starting position. Rest.

Variation I

Lie on your back. Bend one leg; rest the sole of the foot flat on the mat. Raise the other leg; tuck the fingers of both hands under the toes. Slowly straighten the leg. Repeat with the other leg.

Variation II

Called the Partridge, this spread-leg version conditions your inner thigh muscles and contributes to pelvic health.

1 Follow steps 1 to 5 of the instructions for the Toe-Finger Posture (Lying).
2 *Slowly and carefully* spread your legs as far apart as you can *without strain*.
3 Hold the spread-leg posture for as long as you are comfortable in it, breathing regularly.
4 Bring your legs together and slowly resume your starting position. Rest.

Toe-Finger Posture (Sitting)
What it does

The Toe-Finger Posture (Sitting) offers the same benefits as the lying version (Figure 45). Since it is also a balancing exercise, this posture is superb for developing good concentration and coordination. See also the Toe-Finger Posture (Lying).

Variation

In this version of the Toe-Finger Posture (Sitting), you follow steps 1 to 4 of the basic posture, then *slowly and carefully* spread your legs as far apart as you can *without strain*.

Hold the spread-leg posture for as long as you can with absolute comfort while breathing regularly. Resume your starting position. Rest.

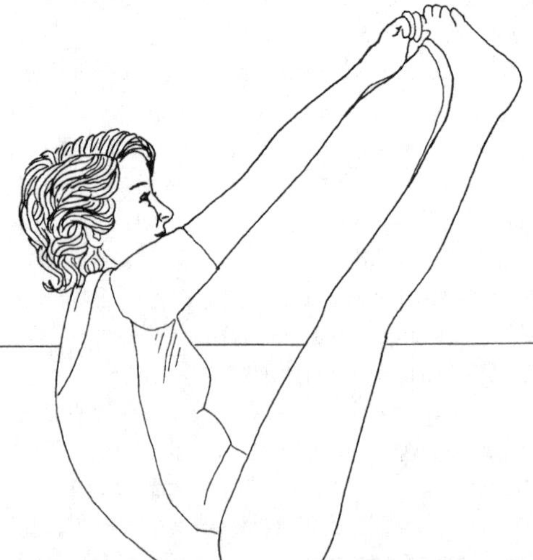

Figure 46 **Toe-Finger Posture (Sitting)**

Toe-Finger Posture (Standing)
What it does
The benefits of practising this posture are the same as for the Toe-Finger Posture (Sitting). See also the Toe-Finger Posture (Lying).

How to do it
1 Stand tall and breathe regularly.
2 Shift your weight onto one foot. Exhale and *carefully* lift the other foot; bring it towards you.
3 Grasp the toes of the raised foot with one or both hands. (If you use one hand, swing the other hand to the side to help you to maintain your balance.)
4 Holding your toes securely, straighten your raised leg, alert for any hint of strain on your hamstring muscles (Figure 47).
5 Stay in the posture for as long as you comfortably can, breathing regularly.
6 Bend your raised leg, release your hold on the toes and return to your starting position.
7 Rest briefly.

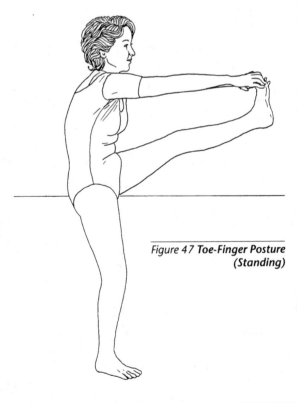

*Figure 47 **Toe-Finger Posture (Standing)***

8 Repeat the exercise (steps 2 to 6), standing on the other foot this time. Rest afterwards.

Variation
1 Stand tall and breathe regularly.
2 Shift your weight onto one foot.
3 Raise the other foot and grasp the toes with one hand only. Swing the other hand sideways to help you to maintain your balance.
4 *Carefully* straighten the raised leg.
5 *Slowly and with control* bring the raised leg to the side, as far as you comfortably can.
6 Hold the posture for as long as you can or are comfortable in it, breathing regularly.
7 *Slowly* bring the raised leg back to the front.
8 *Carefully* resume your starting position. Rest briefly.
9 Repeat the exercise with the other leg (steps 2 to 8).

Note When practising the standing and sitting versions of this posture, fix your gaze on a still object, such as a door handle, a picture on a wall or an ornament, to help you to keep focused and so maintain your balance. Concentrating on your slow, smooth breathing is also useful.

The Tree
What it does
The Tree is a balancing posture. It strengthens the legs and it is excellent for cultivating nerve-muscle coordination and promoting alertness and concentration.

How to do it
1 Stand tall, with your feet together and your arms relaxed at your sides. Breathe regularly.
2 Shift your weight onto one foot. Use your hands to help you to place the sole of the other foot high up against the inside of your opposite thigh.
3 Inhale and raise both arms straight overhead. Press your palms together if you can (Figure 48).
4 Stay in this posture for as long as you comfortably can, breathing regularly.

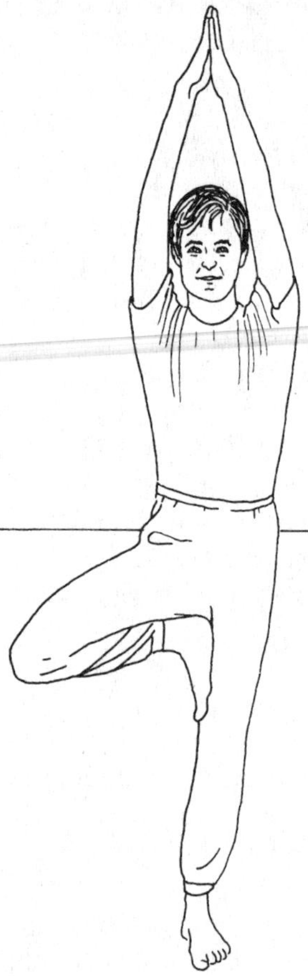

Note To help you to maintain your balance, fix your gaze on a still object in front of you, such as a door handle or a picture on a wall. Keeping your attention focused on your slow, smooth breathing is also useful in helping you to stay steady.

Holy Fig Tree Posture
What it does
Simple though it seems, this posture is surprisingly energizing. It helps to clear respiratory (breathing) passages and improve circulation.

Because it is a balancing exercise, the Holy Fig Tree Posture is excellent for improving concentration and coordination.

How to do it
1 Stand tall. Breathe regularly.
2 Shift your weight onto your right foot. Raise your right arm straight upwards, keeping it alongside your ear.
3 Lift your left foot; point it backwards, keeping the leg as straight as you can. Remain standing tall.
4 Stretch your left arm to the side, at about shoulder level (Figure 49).
5 Hold the posture for as long as you are comfortable in it, breathing regularly.
6 Return to your starting position. Rest.
7 Repeat the exercise (steps 2 to 6), substituting the word 'left' for 'right' and vice versa in the instructions.

Figure 48 *The Tree*

5 Return to your starting position. Rest.
6 Repeat steps 2 to 5, this time balancing on the other foot.

Variations
Fold one leg inwards and use your hands to help you to rest the foot *carefully* against the opposite thigh, as high up as you find comfortable (Half Lotus, Figure 27).

Vary your arm and hand position as follows: stretch your arms sideways, at about shoulder level. Relax your wrists.

Then bring your palms together in front of your chest.

Experiment with combinations of leg and arm positions.

Note Focus your attention on a still object, such as a vase of flowers or a picture on a wall, to help you to maintain your balance. Concentrating on your regular breathing while practising this and other balancing postures is also useful in helping you to stay steady.

Triangle Posture
What it does
The Triangle Posture offers a chance to tone up various muscles that are ordinarily under-exercised. It conditions the muscles of your back and abdomen, improving the muscular supports

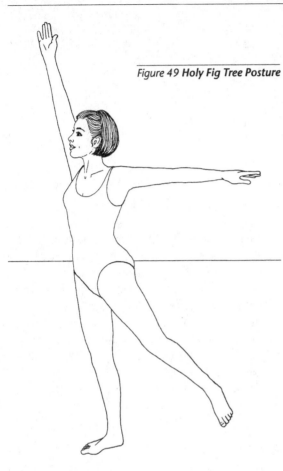

*Figure 49 **Holy Fig Tree Posture***

3 Try to touch your toes with your fingertips. *Do not* lower your head; keep it aligned with your back (Figure 50).

4 Hold the posture for as long as you comfortably can, breathing regularly.

5 Resume your starting position, synchronizing your movement with regular breathing. Rest.

Yoga Sit-Up

What it does

Safer than the conventional 'sit-up' (with feet held down), the Yoga Sit-Up is superb for developing and maintaining strong abdominal muscles. Firm abdominal muscles are important for supporting the back muscles, and are therefore necessary for spinal health.

How to do it

1 Lie on your back, with your legs stretched out in front of you and separated a little. Relax your arms at your sides. Breathe regularly.

2 Bend your knees and slide your feet towards your bottom, until you can rest your feet flat on the mat. Maintain this distance between feet and bottom for the remainder of the exercise.

3 Rest your palms on your thighs.

4 Exhaling, *slowly and carefully* raise your head and shoulders. Keep your eyes fixed on your hands. Slide your hands as if reaching for your

of organs within the abdomen and pelvis. It gently stretches the muscles of your legs and arms, helping to keep them firm.

The Triangle Posture may be difficult for beginners. If at first attempt you find it disheartening, *do not give up*. Continue to practise simpler forwards-bending postures meanwhile, such as the Alternate Leg Stretch (Figure 6), and exercises to loosen tight hamstrings, such as the ankle warm-ups (Chapter 3) and the Dog Stretch (Figure 15), until you become more supple. You can then try this position again, but *do not strain*.

1 Stand tall, with your feet together and your weight equally distributed. Relax your arms at your sides. Breathe regularly.

2 Exhaling, bend forwards at your hips rather than at your waist. Keep your upper body and your legs straight.

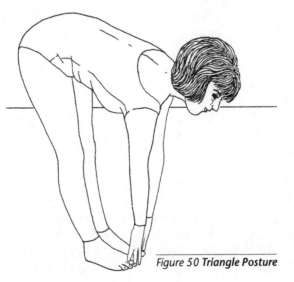

*Figure 50 **Triangle Posture***

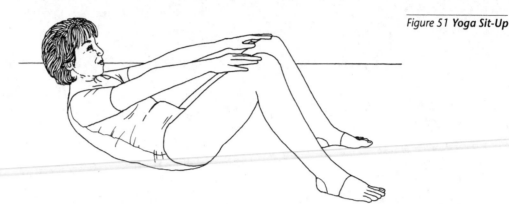

Figure 51 Yoga Sit-Up

knees. When you feel your abdominal muscles tighten as much as you can comfortably tolerate it, stop (Figure 51).

5 Hold the posture for as long as you are comfortable in it, breathing regularly.

6 *Slowly and carefully* curl yourself onto the mat, from bottom to top, until you are again lying flat.

7 Stretch out your legs. Relax your arms and hands at your sides. Rest.

Variation

To do this version of the posture above (called the Diagonal Curl-Up), follow steps 1 and 2 of the basic exercise, but instead of sliding your hands towards your knees, reach for the outside of your right knee.

Hold the posture for as long as you comfortably can while breathing regularly. Return to your starting position. Rest. Repeat the posture on the opposite side (reach for the outside of your left knee). Rest afterwards.

Note In the basic Yoga Sit-Up, it is not necessary to touch your knees. Simply reach for them.

SUGGESTED DAILY PROGRAMMES

Your daily yoga programme, however short, should include certain essential exercises. The following three examples are offered as a guide only. Use them to help you to custom-design *your own* programme, always remembering that you are a unique individual, with your own special needs, strengths and limitations.

The suggested sequences attempt to arrange the exercises in an order that will make the transition from one posture to the next as smooth as possible, and to follow one posture with a counter-posture (for instance, a forwards-bending posture is generally followed by a backwards-bending one). These are examples only. Modify them to suit your particular circumstances.

For Beginners

- **Warm-Ups** Chapter 3. Include: The Butterfly (Figure 1)
- **Sitting Postures** Lotus: Perfect Posture (Figure 26) The Mountain (Figure 29), Squatting Posture (Figure 35)
- **Lying Postures** Knee Press (Figure 24), Pose of Tranquility (Figure 32)
- **Standing Postures** Corrective Prayer Posture (Figure 11)
- **Forwards-Bending Postures** Alternate Leg Stretch (Figure 6), Curling Leaf (Figure 13), Yoga Sit-Up (Figure 51)
- **Backwards-Bending Postures** The Bridge (Figure 8), Chest Expander (Figure 9), The Locust (Figure 25)
- **Sideways-Bending Posture** Half Moon (Figure 20)
- **Twisting Posture** Spinal Twist (Figure 34) and simplified variation

- **Inverted Posture** Dog Stretch (Figure 15)
- **Balance Postures** Dancer's Pose (Figure 14), The Tree (Figure 48)
- **Meditative Exercise** Candle Concentration (Figure 53)
- **Breathing Exercises** Chapter 5

Suggested Sequence

1 Warm-ups – Chapter 3
2 The Mountain – Figure 29
3 Yoga Sit-Up – Figure 51
4 The Bridge – Figure 8
5 Curling Leaf – Figure 13
6 The Locust – Figure 25
7 Knee Press – Figure 24
8 Spinal Twist – Figure 34
9 Dog Stretch – Figure 15
10 Corrective Prayer Posture – Figure 11
11 Half Moon – Figure 20
12 The Tree – Figure 48
13 Squatting Posture – Figure 35
14 Pose of Tranquility – Figure 32
   Breathing Exercises – Chapter 5
   Candle Concentration – Figure 53

INTERMEDIATE LEVEL

- **Warm-Ups** Chapter 3. Include: The Butterfly (Figure 1), Rock-and-Roll (Figure 4) and up to six sets of Sun Salutations (Figures 36–44)
- **Sitting Postures** Lotus: Perfect Posture (Figure 26), Half Lotus (Figure 27), The Mountain (Figure 29), Squatting Posture (Figure 35) and the Toe-Finger Posture, Sitting (Figure 46)
- **Lying Postures** The Fish (Figure 17), Pose of Tranquility (Figure 32), Toe-Finger Posture, Lying (Figure 45)
- **Standing Posture** Corrective Prayer Posture (Figure 11)
- **Forwards-Bending Postures** Curling Leaf (Figure 13), Forwards Bend, Sitting (Figure 18), The Plough (Figure 31), Yoga Sit-Up (Figure 51)
- **Backwards-Bending Postures** Chest Expander (Figure 9), The Locust (Figure 25), Pelvic Stretch (Figure 30)
- **Sideways-Bending Postures** Cross Beam

(Figure 12), Half Moon (Figure 20)
- **Twisting Postures** Spinal Twist (Figure 34) and first two variations
- **Inverted Postures** Half Shoulderstand (Figure 21)
- **Balance Postures** Dancer's Pose (Figure 14) and variation, the Tree (Figure 48) and variation with the leg in Half Lotus position, Holy Tree Fig Posture (Figure 49)
- **Meditative Exercise** Candle Concentration (Figure 53)
- **Breathing Exercises** Chapter 5.

Suggested Sequence

1 Warm-Ups – Chapter 3
2 Forwards Bend, Sitting – Figure 18
3 Pelvic Stretch – Figure 30
4 Curling Leaf – Figure 13
5 Cross Beam – Figure 12
6 Spinal Twist – Figure 34
7 Half Shoulderstand – Figure 21
8 The Plough – Figure 31
9 The Locust – Figure 25
10 Corrective Prayer Posture – Figure 11
11 Holy Fig Tree Posture – Figure 49
12 Squatting Posture – Figure 35
13 Pose of Tranquility – Figure 32
   Breathing Exercises – Chapter 5
   Meditation – Chapter 6

ADVANCED LEVEL

- **Warm-Ups** Chapter 3. Include: The Butterfly (Figure 1) and up to twelve sets of Sun Salutations (Figures 36–44)
- **Sitting Postures** Knee and Thigh Stretch (Figure 23), Half Lotus (Figure 27), Full Lotus (Figure 28), Squatting Posture (Figure 35)
- **Lying Postures** The Fish (Figure 17) and variation with legs folded, Toe-Finger Posture, Lying (Figure 45) and variation, Pose of Tranquility (Figure 32)
- **Forwards-Bending Postures** Curling Leaf (Figure 13), Forwards Bend, Sitting (Figure 18), Forwards Bend, Standing (Figure 19), Knee Press (Figure 24), The Plough (Figure 31), Triangle Posture (Figure 50)

- **Backwards-Bending Postures** The Fish (Figure 17) and the folded-legs variation, Inclined Plane (Figure 22), The Locust (Figure 25) and the advanced variation
- **Sideways-Bending Postures** Cross Beam (Figure 12), Half Moon (Figure 20)
- **Twisting Posture** Spinal Twist (Figure 34), advanced (second) variation
- **Inverted Postures** Half Shoulderstand (Figure 21), The Shoulderstand (Figure 33)
- **Balance Postures** Dancer's Pose (Figure 14), variation, The Eagle (Figure 16) and variation, and the Toe-Finger Posture, Standing (Figure 47)
- **Meditative Exercise** Meditation (chapter 6)
- **Breathing Exercises** Chapter 5.

Suggested Sequence
1 Warm-Ups – Chapter 3
2 Knee and Thigh Stretch – Figure 23
3 Forwards Bend, Sitting – Figure 18
4 Inclined Plane – Figure 22
5 Knee Press – Figure 24
6 Half Shoulderstand – Figure 21
7 The Shoulderstand – Figure 33
8 The Plough – Figure 31
9 The Fish – Figure 17
10 Knee Press – Figure 24
11 The Locust – Figure 25
12 Curling Leaf – Figure 13
13 Cross Beam – Figure 12
14 Spinal Twist – Figure 34
15 Corrective Prayer Posture – Figure 11
16 The Eagle – Figure 16
17 Pose of Tranquillity – Figure 32
Breathing Exercises – Chapter 5
Meditation – Chapter 6

5

BREATHING EXERCISES

Respiratory function is one of the best indicators of biological age. Although you may be sixty years of age chronologically, you may in fact have the physiology of a forty-year-old if your breathing apparatus, or lungs, are in peak condition.

Lung function tends to diminish with age, partly because of changes in the structure of the rib-cage and chest muscles, and indeed in the lungs themselves. It is further decreased by disease and harmful forms of stress. But there is a bright side to this gloomy prospect: Nature has given us the resources to deal effectively with these changes, and a measure of control over the breathing process. By practising yoga breathing exercises every day, you will be able to keep your respiratory system in the best possible working order. This will increase your potential for living longer and more fully, and for looking and feeling youthful.

RESPIRATION AND CIRCULATION

Respiration is the act of breathing and consists of two movements: inhalation and exhalation. In quiet breathing most of the work is done by the diaphragm, a dome-shaped muscle that separates the chest and abdominal cavities.

When you *inhale*, the diaphragm contracts and causes the chest to enlarge from top to bottom. At the same time the chest widens from back to front and from side to side as its muscles contract. When this occurs, the lungs expand to fill the increased space, and air is drawn into them through the air passages.

When you *exhale*, air is pushed out as the muscles relax, and also by the elastic recoil of the lungs.

The primary work of the lungs is to transfer oxygen to the blood and remove carbon dioxide. Oxygen combines with haemoglobin (the colouring matter of red blood cells) and is carried to all the cells so that they can carry out vital functions. Carbon dioxide, which is a metabolic waste product, is removed from the blood during exhalation.

Respiration and blood circulation work very closely together. Inhaled air, which contains oxygen, passes through the air passages into the lungs. The oxygen is transferred to the blood. The heart pumps this oxygen-rich blood to every part of the body through a network of blood vessels.

After blood has circulated throughout the body, it returns to the heart greatly depleted of oxygen. It is then pumped again through the lungs where it picks up oxygen and the whole process repeats itself continuously.

BENEFITS OF YOGA

Yoga breathing exercises are collectively referred to as *pranayama*, a work taken from Sanskrit. 'Prana' means 'vital breath' and has connotations of vitality and even life itself. Pranayama refers to the integration of the nervous and respiratory systems.

Changes of feeling are reflected in patterns of breathing. Fear, for example, produces fast, shallow breathing. Anger results in short, quick inhalations and strong, rapid exhalations. In anxiety states, breathing is also fast and sometimes irregular. Emotions such as happiness, love and forgiveness, on the other hand, induce slow, smooth, even respirations and a general feeling of well-being.

The reverse is also true: consciously changing the pattern of breathing will bring about a change in emotional state. I vividly remember sitting beside a young patient, in the early hours of the morning, painstakingly instructing her in a breathing technique to counteract a panic attack. The technique we used was the Anti-Anxiety Breath, which is described later in this chapter, and it worked very well indeed. Within minutes, the young woman had regained considerable calm and was able to return to bed and to sleep until it was time for breakfast.

You can, in a similar way, use your breath to very good advantage as an effective stress management tool.

Regular practice of yoga breathing exercises helps you to develop good breathing habits, thus increasing your chances of a long and productive life. It helps you to become more aware, alert and in control of yourself. Proper breathing can increase the availability of oxygen to the body's cells. It is like an internal massage; it relaxes muscles, improves blood flow and reduces cramps and other discomforts.

Diaphragmatic breathing (as opposed to shallow breathing, using mostly the chest muscles) exposes the lower lobes of the lungs, which have a rich blood supply, to a good blast of oxygen. The blood then picks up the oxygen to feed the rest of the body. Diaphragmatic breathing, moreover, enhances the elimination of wastes by squeezing more stale air out of the system than chest breathing does. In short, it improves circulation and decreases the heart's work-load.

Regularly practised, yoga breathing exercises strengthen other parts of your respiratory system. They bring your sympathetic and para-sympathetic nervous systems into balance, thereby producing a calming effect, since breath and the emotions are intimately linked. They can also help to reduce cravings for food, alcohol and nicotine. In addition, the exercises can strengthen the immune system, giving you reinforced protection against disease. They can help, as well, to normalize body weight and increase energy levels.

Innumerable forces are at work to influence the way we live and breathe. Two examples that come to mind immediately are stress and environmental pollutants. But we have the means by which to counteract these agents and we carry it with us wherever we go: our breath.

PREPARING FOR THE EXERCISES

Before your practise yoga breathing exercises, there are several points to note:

1 Maintain good posture. Hold your spine naturally erect but not rigid. This will relax your rib-cage and prevent compression of your lungs and other vital structures.
2 When you inhale, do so slowly, smoothly and deeply, using your diaphragm as a sort of suction pump and your chest muscles to expand your rib-cage. Breathe through your nostrils (with your mouth closed, unless otherwise instructed), to warm, moisten and filter the air.
3 When you exhale, do so slowly, steadily and thoroughly, using your diaphragm as a sort of squeezing pump.

4 Keep your body as relaxed as possible, paying special attention to your jaws, face and hands.
5 Keep your breathing rhythm regular, unless otherwise instructed. *Do not hold your breath.*

Before you start the exercises, attend also to the following:

- Empty your bladder, and your bowel if possible. Clean your teeth and tongue. Clear your nostrils as follows:
- Fill a cupped hand with warm water. Close one nostril. *Gently* sniff a little of the water into the other nostril and then briskly expel it. Repeat this once or twice. Repeat the procedure with the other nostril.

You may practise the breathing exercises about fifteen minutes after practising yoga postures. Afterwards, lie down and relax, as in the Pose of Tranquility (Figure 32).

Finally, *avoid* practising yoga postures immediately after a session of breathing exercises.

THE EXERCISES

Cautions *Omit* the Bellows Breath if you have a heart condition, high blood-pressure, epilepsy, a hernia or an ear or eye disorder. *See also* Chapter 2 for general cautions.

Alternate Nostril Breathing
What it does
Alternate Nostril Breathing is a technique that stimulates the inner lining of the nostrils by alternating the air flow and sending sequential impulses to the two brain hemispheres.

Modern research has revealed that these two hemispheres have different functions: the left chiefly influences language and mathematical skills while the right controls imaginative and intuitive functions, such as spatial orientation and creative thinking.

Alternate Nostril Breathing helps to integrate the functions of both hemispheres, with resulting integration of mind and body, and greater mental and physical energy. It is also a very soothing exercise. It helps to assuage anxiety, which can aggravate pain and various other physical discomforts. It is, in addition, a useful antidote for sleeplessness.

How to do it
1 Sit tall, in any comfortable position. Relax your jaws. Relax the rest of your body. Breathe regularly.
2 Rest your left hand in your lap, on your knee or on the armrest of a chair, depending on where you are sitting.
3 Arrange the fingers of your right hand as follows: fold the two middle fingers inwards towards the palm (or you may rest them lightly on the bridge of your nose); use your thumb to close your right nostril once the exercise is in progress, and your ring finger (or ring and little fingers) to close your left nostril (Figure 52).

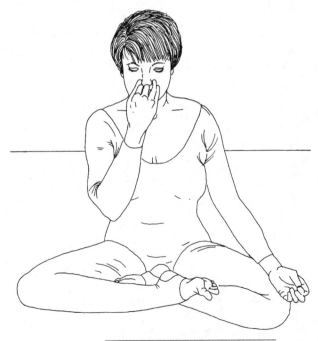

Figure 52 *Alternate Nostril Breathing*

4 Close your eyes and begin: close your right nostril and inhale slowly, smoothly and deeply as you can *without strain* through your left nostril.

5 Close your left nostril and release closure of your right; exhale.

6 Inhale through your right nostril.

7 Close your right nostril; release closure of your left and exhale.

This completes one round of Alternate Nostril Breathing.

8 Repeat steps 4 to 7 in smooth succession as many times as you wish, until you feel a sense of calm and well-being.

9 Relax your right arm and hand. Resume regular breathing. Open your eyes.

Anti-Anxiety Breath

What it does

Excellent for counteracting anxiety, this breathing exercise is also very useful for coping with other stressful emotions such as apprehension, frustration and anger. For a panic attack, it is a technique without equal. You can help someone in such a crisis by clearly and patiently instructing him or her to practise steps 2 to 4 again and again until calm has been restored.

How to do it

1 Sit tall. Close your eyes or keep them open. Relax your jaws. (You may also practise this exercise while lying or standing.)

2 Inhale quietly through your nostrils – slowly, smoothly and as deeply as possible without strain.

3 Exhale steadily through your nostrils, focusing your attention on your upper abdomen, near your navel.

4 Before inhaling again, mentally count 'one thousand', 'two thousand'. (This helps to lengthen your exhalation and prevent rapid breathing.)

5 Repeat steps 2 to 4 again and again, in smooth succession, until you feel calm.

6 Resume regular breathing.

Note Combine imagery with this exercise, if you wish. Visualize filling your system with positive things such as courage, patience and hope as you inhale. As you exhale, imagine sending away on the outgoing breath negative things such as fear, sadness and disappointment.

Bellows Breath

Caution *Do not* practise this exercise if you have a heart condition, high blood-pressure, epilepsy, a hernia, or an ear or eye disorder. Practise the Cleansing Breath instead.

What it does

The Bellows Breath is excellent for cleansing the respiratory passages. It stimulates lung tissues, and gently yet effectively massages abdominal organs. It thus helps to improve elimination. It is also superb for strengthening the diaphragm and the chest and abdominal muscles, and trains you to control your exhalation, a skill that is useful for those who suffer from asthma. In addition, the Bellows Breath revitalizes the nervous system.

How to do it

1 Sit comfortably. Relax your arms and hands. Close your eyes or keep them open. Relax your jaws. Breathe regularly. (You may also practise this exercise standing or lying.)

2 Inhale slowly, smoothly and as deeply as you can without strain.

3 Exhale briskly as if sneezing, focusing your attention on your abdomen which will tighten and flatten.

4 Inhalation will follow almost involuntarily as you relax your abdomen and chest.

5 Repeat steps 3 and 4 again and again, in rapid succession. (If you think of a bellows collapsing and expanding, it will help you with your technique.)

6 Practise the Bellows Breath for several seconds to begin with. Gradually extend practice time as your stamina increases and you become more familiar with the exercise.

7 Resume regular breathing.

Note This exercise is a good way to start a session of breathing exercises. Practise it outdoors whenever you can, to take advantage of the fresh air.

Breathing Away Pain
What it does
Breathing and emotions are closely linked. By consciously slowing down your respirations you become less tense. As tension decreases, circulation to a painful area improves and pain-producing irritants are eliminated. In addition, focusing on the breathing process itself diverts your attention temporarily, and your awareness of pain is lessened.

Use this technique, duly modified, to 'breathe away fatigue' and other unwelcome states such as resentment and perceived hurts.

How to do it
1 Sit or lie comfortably. Close your eyes. Relax your jaws and breathe regularly.
2 Rest your hands lightly on the painful area and make this the focus of your attention. As you take a long, steady breath inwards, visualize a soothing jet of water flowing through your hands into the affected part. Imagine that the water has healing properties.
3 Breathe out slowly and steadily, visualizing an outpouring of irritants and impurities.
4 Repeat steps 2 and 3 again and again, in smooth succession, until your experience relief.
5 Relax your arms and hands. Breathe regularly.

Note Use whatever imagery you prefer or feel more comfortable with. For example, you may visualize a gentle, healing light or a soothing lotion entering the painful area on inhalation; or imagine pain-producing deposits floating away on the outgoing breath. Modify the exercise to suit your special needs.

Cleansing Breath
What it does
The Cleansing Breath is a wonderful technique for releasing pent-up emotion and for managing stress. Practise it whenever you feel tension mounting, or whenever you feel anxious or frustrated.

How to do it
1 Sit comfortably. Relax your arms and hands. Close your eyes or keep them open. Breathe regularly. (You may also practise this exercise standing or lying.)
2 Inhale through your nostrils slowly, smoothly and as deeply as you can without strain.
3 Exhale through pouted lips, as if whistling or cooling a hot drink. Do so slowly and smoothly.
4 When your exhalation is complete, close your lips and repeat steps 2 and 3 again and again in smooth succession, until you feel calmer and more in control of yourself.
5 Resume regular breathing.

Note With appropriate modifications, you can practise the Cleansing Breath wherever you feel comfortable doing so, such as while driving in difficult traffic conditions, before an interview or during or after a crisis.

Complete Breath
What it does
This exercise trains you to use your diaphragm and other structures involved in respiration in the most advantageous way possible (*see* the section in benefits earlier in this chapter).

How to do it
1 Sit comfortably. Relax your arms and hands. Close your eyes or keep them open. Breathe regularly. (You may also practise this exercise standing or lying.)
2 Inhale through your nostrils slowly, smoothly and as deeply as possible without strain. Pay attention to the movement of your rib-cage,

which will expand, and to your abdomen, which will rise.

3 Exhale slowly, steadily and thoroughly, again focusing on your chest, which will now relax, and your abdomen, which will flatten.

4 Repeat steps 2 and 3 again and again in smooth succession for a minute to start with. Increase practice time as you become more comfortable with the exercise.

5 Resume regular breathing.

Notes When first attempting the Complete Breath, you may find the following useful, to help you to appreciate the respiratory process:

- Place your palms lightly against your abdomen near your navel, with the middle finger of one hand touching that of the other. As you inhale, the fingers will separate and as you exhale they will meet again.
- Try doing the Complete Breath as you lie on your abdomen, with your head turned to the side. Put a flat cushion or folded towel under your hips to avoid straining your back.
- Incorporate visualization into the exercise: as you inhale, imagine filling your system with positive things such as peace, love and hope. As you exhale, imagine sending away on the outgoing breath negative influences such as self-doubt, sorrow and hatred.
- If you are unclear as to whether your abdomen should rise or fall as you breathe in or out, think of a balloon: as you put air into it, it becomes larger; as you let the air out, it collapses. Use the following mnemonic: 'Air in, abdomen fat. Air out, abdomen flat.'

Cooling Breath
What it does
When your body is overheated, such as when you have a fever or the weather is hot, the Cooling Breath is a useful exercise for restoring comfort.

How to do it
1 Sit naturally erect. Relax your arms and hands. Close your eyes or keep them open. Breathe regularly. (You may also practise this exercise standing or lying.)

2 Stick out your tongue and curl it lengthways to form a sort of tube. Inhale slowly and steadily through this 'tube'.

3 Pull in your tongue and close your mouth. Exhale slowly and steadily through your nostrils.

4 Repeat steps 2 and 3 again and again in smooth succession, as many times as you wish.

5 Breathe regularly.

Humming Breath
What it does
The Humming Breath is, in effect, a meditation on sound. It calms the mind, soothes the spirit and relaxes the body.

How to do it
1 Sit comfortably. Relax your arms and hands. Close your eyes. Unclench your teeth to relax your jaws. Close, but do not compress, your lips. Breathe regularly.

2 Inhale slowly, smoothly and as deeply as you can without strain.

3 As you exhale slowly and steadily, make a humming sound like that of a bee. The humming should last as long as the exhalation does.

4 Repeat steps 2 and 3 again and again in smooth succession, until you feel calm.

5 Resume regular breathing.

Notes Practise the Humming Breath after a hectic day, when you need a few minutes of solitude to restore your perspective on life and regain a measure of self-control. Practise it when you feel troubled, to relax and comfort you.

Give full attention to both the breathing and to the humming. This is what pulls your thoughts away from disturbing environmental stimuli and helps to re-establish balance.

Sighing Breath
What it does
When your chest is so tight that you are unable to take a deep breath, the Sighing Breath is the exercise of choice. It relaxes not only tense chest muscles but also the whole body. Practise it any time you feel under pressure.

How to do it
1 Sit comfortably. Relax your arms and hands. Close your eyes or keep them open. Relax your jaws.
2 Take two, three or more quick inward sniffs, as if breaking up an inhalation into small parts.
3 Exhale slowly and steadily through your nostrils.
4 Repeat steps 2 and 3 several times, until you feel your chest relaxing and you can then take one deep inward breath without straining.
5 Resume regular breathing.

Walking Breath
What it does
This exercise, generally practised outdoors, calms the nerves and helps to revitalize both body and mind.

How to do it
1 Hold yourself tall but not stiff. Relax your jaws and breathe regularly.
2 As you begin to walk, inhale slowly, smoothly and as deeply as you can without strain, for the duration of two, three, four or more steps.
3 Exhale slowly and steadily for the duration of two, three, four or more steps, according to what is most comfortable for you.
4 Repeat steps 2 and 3 again and again in smooth succession, for a minute or two to begin with. Increase the time spent practising the exercise, as suits you.
5 Breathe regularly for the rest of your walk.

Notes Practise this exercise for only a small part of your walk at first. This allows your lungs time to accommodate to what may be an unaccustomed intake of oxygen all at once. Too much oxygen intake too quickly may produce dizziness. As your stamina builds up, however, you can increase the number of steps per inhalation and exhalation. Try to make the exhalation a little longer than the inhalation, to ensure thorough elimination of stale air.

Whispering Breath
What it does
The Whispering Breath is an excellent exercise to practise if you suffer from asthma or have any other disorder that limits respiratory function. It also helps to improve concentration and it promotes general relaxation.

How to do it
You will need a lighted candle when first learning to do this exercise.
1 Sit comfortably in front of a lighted candle. Relax your arms and hands. Relax your jaws. Breathe regularly.
2 Inhale slowly, smoothly and steadily through your nostrils.
3 Through pouted lips *very slowly, gently and with control*, blow at the candle flame and make it flicker, but *not* to put it out.
4 Close your mouth when your exhalation is complete and repeat steps 2 and 3 again and again in smooth succession.
5 When you feel tired, end the exercise and rest. Resume regular breathing.

Notes When you have mastered this exercise, you can dispense with the candle. Close your eyes and imagine that you are blowing at a flame. Try practising the Whispering Breath lying, standing or walking up one or more flights of stairs.

6

MENTAL EXERCISES

When you practise the exercises in Chapters 3 and 4, you are practising both physical and mental exercises. Along with the stretching synchronized with breathing, you are focusing your attention on every move you make, shutting out any activity or thought that is not pertinent. You are therefore practising concentration and an active form of meditation. This chapter introduces you to more passive forms of meditation, in which you are required to sit still rather than move parts of your body. The postures and other exercises you practise will prepare you well for what follows.

MEDITATION

Meditation is a natural tool for relaxing your conscious mind without clouding your awareness. Doctors describe this state as 'hypometabolic wakefulness', which means that metabolism has decreased even though you are still conscious and awake. Doctors also refer to the meditative state as one of 'restful alertness', a term that is seemingly contradictory.

When you are asleep, for instance, your heartbeat slows down, oxygen consumption decreases and consciousness fades. When you are awake, on the other hand, your heartbeat is faster, oxygen consumption increases and you are usually alert. During meditation these opposite states are united, so that although your body becomes deeply relaxed, your mind remains awake and alert.

BENEFITS OF MEDITATION
Early in this century, researchers discovered that long-term meditation actually helped to decrease a person's metabolic age. Subjects who had been meditating for fewer than five years had an average biological age of five years younger than they were chronologically. Subjects who had been meditating for more than five years had an average biological age of twelve years younger than their chronological age. Subsequent research confirmed these findings: people who meditated regularly visited doctors and were admitted to hospitals only half as often as those who did not meditate. They also had a lower incidence of heart disease and cancer. One of the most remarkable discoveries on the value of regular meditation, with regard to ageing, was that meditators aged 65 years and over showed the most improvement in health status.

People who meditate regularly tend to have higher DHEA levels than those who do not. DHEA, or dehydroepiandrosterone, is a substance secreted by the cortex (external layer) of the adrenal glands. DHEA levels peak about the age of 25 years and decline as we grow older.

DHEA is a precursor (forerunner) of stress hormones. Every time the body makes these hormones, it uses up some DHEA, which accounts for its decrease over a lifetime. High DHEA levels are associated with a lower incidence of breast cancer, coronary artery disease and osteoporosis, and longer survival from all diseases in older men.

The obvious inference to be drawn from the above is that if you can prevent your DHEA levels from declining too rapidly, you can retard ageing through effective stress management. In fact, people who are long-term meditators show less biological ageing than non-meditators, independent of factors such as alcohol consumption, diet and weight.

Regular meditation practice helps to counteract deep-rooted tensions so that you become more at ease with yourself and with others. This results in greater self-confidence and enhanced productivity. It also contributes to a heightened sense of self-control, so that things which were previously perceived as insurmount-able now begin to seem at least manageable.

Meditation is truly nature's tranquillizer. You can help yourself by meditating before a public appearance, a surgical procedure, an interview or any other event in which you anticipate difficulty or distress.

Increasingly, doctors are recommending a period or two of daily meditation as an adjunct to treatment for various health disorders including heart disease, high blood-pressure, migraine headaches, stomach and intestinal ulcers and various nervous system conditions. Daily meditation may also be practised as a preventive measure. Before starting to practise meditation, however, be sure to *check with your doctor*.

HOW IT WORKS

During meditation, both the consumption of oxygen and the elimination of the waste product carbon dioxide decrease markedly, but there is no alteration in their balance. This indicates that the circulatory system is functioning effectively. During meditation, the heart's work-load is decreased and the heartbeat and breathing rates slow down. This indicates a state of deep relaxation.

Skin resistance increases significantly during meditation, denoting a calm emotional state. Metabolic rate drops by about 20 per cent, with a corresponding fall in blood-pressure. Lactate ion concentration (suspected of affecting both emotional state and muscle tone adversely) decreases by about 33 per cent. Brainwave recordings on an EEG (electro-encephalograph) show an unusual abundance of alpha waves, implying that the brain is alert yet wonderfully rested.

PREPARING FOR MEDITATION

An important prerequisite for meditating successfully is the ability to sit still for about twenty uninterrupted minutes. It is therefore worthwhile trying to master the Lotus postures (Figures 26 to 28) and the Pose of Tranquillity (Figure 32). If you find the folded-legs seated postures uncomfortable, you may sit on a chair. Regular practice of the breathing exercises will train you in the art of sitting relaxed and maintaining good posture for increasingly long periods of time.

Always meditate before, rather than after, a meal to prevent the process of digestion from interfering with concentration.

Choose a quiet place in which to meditate. Arrange for twenty minutes of uninterrupted time.

Sit comfortably, with your spine in good alignment and supported if necessary. Rest your hands in your lap, on your knees or on the arm-rest of a chair. Close your eyes. Relax your body from head to toes. Breathe regularly.

Try to meditate at least once a day, but preferably twice. Start with five or ten minutes, gradually increasing the time to twenty minutes a session.

Candle Concentration
What it does
Candle Concentration is a good way to prepare yourself for daily meditation on a regular basis. Regularly practised, it helps to improve concentration and promote relaxation. It is a good pre-sleep exercise for those who suffer from insomnia. It also strengthens the eyes.

How to do it
Place a lighted candle at or slightly below eye level, on a table, stool or similar prop.

1 Sit tall, in any comfortable position. Relax your hands. Breathe regularly. Look intently at the candle flame (Figure 53). Blink if necessary. Spend about a minute on this step, to begin with.
2 Close your eyes and visualize the candle flame. Try to retain the image or to recall it if it vanishes. Spend about a minute on this step, to begin with.

   Do not be anxious if the flame disappears. Mentally try to persuade it to return. If it does not, try the exercise again, from the beginning. Remember to keep breathing regularly.

3 Open your eyes and repeat the exercise (steps 1 to 3), or return to your usual activities.

   With each subsequent exercise session, increase the time spent looking at the candle flame and the time spent recalling its image.

Variation
Instead of a candle, you may use any small, pleasing object, such as a flower, a fruit, a design or even a stone on the beach on which to concentrate.

A Simple Meditation
1 Sit comfortably. Close your eyes. Relax your body. Breathe regularly.
2 Inhale slowly and smoothly through your nostrils.
3 As you exhale slowly and smoothly through your nostrils, mentally say the word 'one'.
4 Repeat steps 2 and 3 again and again in smooth succession.

   If your thoughts stray, guide them back patiently to both the breathing and the repetition of 'one'. Do not be discouraged if this occurs frequently at first. With regular practice, your ability to remain one-pointed will improve.

   When you are ready to end your period of meditation, do so slowly: open your eyes and gently stretch and/or massage your limbs. Never come out of meditation suddenly.

Notes You may substitute any word or short phrase for 'one'. Particularly effective is something related to your religion. Other suggestions are: peace, calm, relax; I feel calm; love and light; nothing can harm me.

   When you are faced with a challenging or perplexing situation, try to recapture the peace you experienced during meditation. It will help you to delay your response somewhat: to act rather than react to unpleasant stimuli. It will provide you with a focal point which will help you to maintain a certain detachment and give you a measure of control. It will also help you to re-establish your equilibrium.

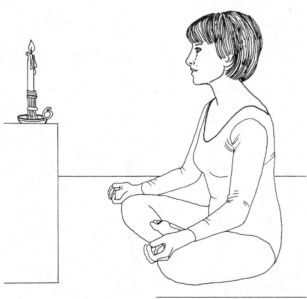

*Figure 53 **Candle Concentration***

Check your breathing periodically to make sure that it is slow and smooth.

A Touch Meditation

You will need a small object that you can hold comfortably in your hands. An ornament, a teacup, a fruit or a small book of devotions or poetry are examples.

1 Sit comfortably. Close your eyes. Relax your body. Breathe regularly.
2 Inhale slowly and smoothly through your nostrils.
3 Exhale slowly and smoothly through your nostrils and focus your attention on the object in your hands.
4 Repeat steps 2 and 3 again and again in smooth succession, using each exhalation to enhance your awareness of the object you are holding, and your sense of touch.

If your thoughts wander, gently re-direct them to both the breathing and the object held. With time and patience, your attention will drift less and less.

End your meditation slowly and with awareness. Do not rush.

Meditation on Sound

The Humming Breath, which is described in Chapter 5, is appropriate for meditating on sound.

A Healing Meditation

The Breathing Away Pain exercise described in Chapter 5 may be used for healing purposes. Simply modify it to suit your special needs, using appropriate imagery and mental suggestion.

A Visualization

1 Sit comfortably. Close your eyes. Relax your body. Breathe regularly.
2 Imagine lying in a meadow early on a deliciously warm day. The grass is soft beneath you. Overhead, fluffy white clouds drift by. The delicate fragrance of wild flowers delights your sense of smell. A meadow lark breaks into joyful song. A gentle breeze caresses your face and arms. Your troubles become a hazy memory. Your frustrations disappear. You feel light and free as a wonderful sense of bliss sweeps over you. This moment is yours to keep and to recapture mentally whenever the need arises.

Savour this pastoral visualization to the full. When you are ready to return to your usual activities, stretch your limbs in a leisurely way. Open your eyes. Get up slowly and carefully.

Notes The above is only one example of therapeutic imagery. There are many possibilities. You can transport yourself mentally to a beach, a mountain glen or a flower garden, and immerse yourself in the touch, smells, sounds and even taste generated by the specific scene. Although it is not yet fully understood how these visualizations work, research has demonstrated the tranquillizing and healing power of such attractive mental images.

7

EATING FOR LONGEVITY

How long we live, and how healthy our lives are, is not determined by heredity alone. Although the genetic code for any trait contains a set of specific instructions, the manner in which these are carried out depends on the nature of their interaction with other sets of instructions and also on their environments. Our genetic constitution is capable of being influenced, and so we should not think that the length of our life is predetermined.

Just as advances in disease control and living conditions have resulted in increased life expectancy for many people, so too has improved nutrition. Better education has given us, for example, knowledge of foods that fight infection and give protection against life-shortening diseases such as cancer and against environmental pollutants. It is largely what we take into our body in the food we eat and the fluids we drink that affects our natural defences (the immune system), and builds and maintains health. Nutrients from an adequate, wholesome diet are processed by the digestive system and transported to every cell, tissue and organ by means of our circulatory system. There is no doubt that our basic genetic inheritance can be helped by rational principles of living, which include good nutrition.

Repairing the body and maintaining good health into advanced age are often slow processes; seldom as fast and dramatic as preventing the spread of infection with antibiotics, for instance, yet much more rapid than was formerly believed. Research has confirmed that we can enhance the functioning of all our body's systems, and in some cases prevent problems from arising, through the intelligent application of sound nutritional principles. To help you to do this, I offer information in this chapter on essential nutrients and food sources from which they can be obtained. Please bear in mind, however, that *all nutrients work together*, and that no single one of them should be viewed as a panacea.

Metabolism slows down as we age and so generally we need less energy (i.e. fewer calories) from our food, depending of course on the nature of our activities. Nevertheless, we continue to need vitamins, minerals and other nutrients. The challenge, then, is to obtain all these from fewer calories, to avoid putting on weight that could prove unhealthy.

If you are considering taking nutritional supplements, it would be prudent to consult a dietitian, nutritionist or other qualified health professional first.

ESSENTIAL NUTRIENTS

WATER

Water is the principal constituent of body fluids. It is the medium by which nutrients are transported to all cells and wastes removed from the system. It is a lubricant and a shock absorber, and essential for preventing the spinal discs (which cushion the bones making up the spine) from drying out as we age. It is necessary for proper digestion, for regulating body temperature, for helping to prevent constipation, bladder infection and dehydration, which is a major cause of preventable ageing.

You can obtain water from all drinkable liquids, but unsweetened fruit and vegetable juices, herbal teas and other non-caffeinated beverages, soups, milk (and, of course, plain tap or mineral water) are among the best sources. Ordinarily, six to eight glasses a day is considered adequate; thirst is not regarded as a good indicator of fluid needs.

FIBRE

Studies have shown that the incidence of disorders such as colitis, colon cancer, haemorrhoids, varicose veins and constipation is much lower among people whose diet is high in fibre than among the general population in industrialized nations. Fibre, moreover, binds cholesterol and prevents its absorption, and is therefore useful in controlling conditions such as atherosclerosis.

Good sources of dietary fibre include bread and other products made from whole grains; fresh fruits and raw vegetables, nuts and legumes (dried peas, beans and lentils).

PROTEIN

Protein forms the basic structure of all cells and is essential for the synthesis of collagen, the 'glue' that holds the cells together. Your hair, skin, nails, eyes and muscles are made of protein.

There are basically two types of protein: complete, which is obtainable from foods of animal origin such as meat, cheese, eggs, milk, poultry and seafood, and which has a proper balance of the eight essential amino acids (protein building-blocks); and incomplete protein, which lacks certain essential amino acids and includes foods such as grains, legumes, nuts and seeds. In certain combinations, however, they can be rendered complete. Examples are: rice and legumes; baked beans and wholewheat bread, and corn and beans.

FAT

Fat is needed to provide energy, conserve heat, produce hormones and help cells to function normally. It supports and protects organs such as the eyes and kidneys and it furnishes EFAs (essential fatty acids). It also provides a vehicle for the transportation of natural fat-soluble vitamins (A, D, E and K).

Good sources of fat include butter, cheese, eggs, milk, nuts, and also oils from vegetables, nuts and seeds such as avocados, olives, peanuts, sunflower and sesame seeds.

COMPLEX CARBOHYDRATES

Complex carbohydrates, in contrast with simple carbohydrates such as refined white rice and sugar, are released slowly from the stomach. They are rich in nutrients, and they provide bulk which appeases appetite and counteracts constipation. They help to prevent overweight and high blood-pressure, and they also aid in lowering elevated blood cholesterol.

Good sources of complex carbohydrates include wholegrain breads and pasta, fresh fruits, and fresh corn and other vegetables.

VITAMINS
Vitamin A

Vitamin A is an antioxidant, that is, it prevents or inhibits oxidation. Important for building resistance to infection, it is also necessary for healthy eyes and good eyesight. It is needed for the normal production of prostate gland fluid, and for the proper repair of bones and connective tissue. In addition, vitamin A is essential for preserving the health of skin, hair, teeth, gums and mucous membranes (which line body cavities and tubular organs).

Vitamin A occurs in two forms: preformed vitamin A (called retinol), which is found in foods of animal origin; and provitamin A (known as carotene), which is provided by foods of both plant and animal origin.

Good vitamin A sources include fresh vegetables, especially intensely green and yellow ones, such as broccoli and carrots, and fresh fruits, especially apricots, cantaloupe melons, papaya and peaches; also milk, milk products and fish liver oils.

The B vitamins

Known as 'the nerve vitamins', this complex of more than twenty vitamins is essential for maintaining a healthy nervous system and for helping to counteract the effects of stress. The B vitamins help to prevent and fight infections and to maintain the health of the skin, hair and nails.

B vitamins may be obtained from brewer's yeast, various fresh fruits and vegetables, green leafy vegetables, legumes, liver, eggs, milk, nuts, seeds, wheatgerm and whole grains and cereals. They are also synthesized by intestinal bacteria.

Following are some notes on individual B vitamins, but please be aware that they *all* work together:

- *Vitamin B_1 (Thiamine)*
  Known as 'the morale vitamin', vitamin B_1 improves mental state and keeps the nervous system, the muscles and the heart functioning normally. It aids appetite and is also needed for proper digestion and sugar utilization. It is useful in combating travel sickness.

- *Vitamin B_2 (Riboflavin)*
  Vitamin B_2 functions with other substances to metabolize proteins, fats and carbohydrates. It aids vision and relieves eye fatigue. It helps to prevent sore lips, mouth and tongue, and it is necessary for healthy skin, hair and nails.

- *Vitamin B_3 (Niacin, Nicotinic Acid, Nicotinamide)*
  Vitamin B_3 is an antioxidant, that is, it helps to prevent or inhibit oxidation. It helps to keep the digestive system healthy, and is necessary for proper sugar utilization. It is important for good circulation and for healthy skin. It helps to prevent bad breath and dizziness, and is useful in the healing of canker sores.

- *Vitamin B_5 (Pantothenic Acid, Pantothenol, Calcium Pantothenate)*
  Vitamin B_5 is necessary to keep the immune system healthy. It helps to maintain a sound nervous system and is useful in preventing fatigue. It helps wounds to heal, and it counteracts skin inflammations. It is also important for the normal functioning of the adrenal glands, which play a vital role in stress reactions.

- *Vitamin B_6 (Pyridoxine)*
  Vitamin B_6 is necessary for maintaining good resistance to disease, for the production of hormones, and for the proper assimilation of protein and fat.

  Other vitamin B_6 roles include: preventing various skin disorders, counteracting nausea, reducing leg cramps, nocturnal muscle spasms, numbness of the hands and certain nerve inflammations of the extremities, promoting the synthesis of anti-ageing nucleic acids, combating depression and acting as a natural diuretic (an agent that increases the secretion of urine).

- *Vitamin B_9 (Folate, Folacin, Folic Acid)*
  Vitamin B_9 helps to prevent anaemia and canker sores, and plays an important role in keeping the immune system functioning effectively. It acts as a pain reliever, and it keeps the skin healthy. Good supplies of folic acid are essential in the early stages of pregnancy for the healthy formation of the baby.

Vitamin B$_9$ may delay the greying of hair when used in conjunction with vitamin B$_5$ and PABA (another B vitamin). It also helps to improve appetite when one is feeling debilitated.

- *Vitamin B$_{12}$ (Cobalamin, Cyano-cobalamin)*
  Essential for the production and regeneration of red blood cells, vitamin B$_{12}$ also helps to maintain the health of the nervous system, and to improve memory, concentration and balance. It is also important for the proper utilization of protein and carbohydrates, and in addition may have a regulating effect on the immune system.

  Vitamin B$_{12}$ is synthesized by intestinal bacteria.

- *Vitamin B$_{15}$ (Pangamic Acid)*
  Vitamin B$_{15}$ extends the lifespan of cells, helps to lower elevated blood cholesterol levels and to relieve chest pain and asthma. It protects against pollutants, counteracts the craving for alcohol and helps to ward off hangovers. It also helps to combat fatigue, stimulate immune responses and promote protein synthesis.

- *Biotin (Coenzyme R, Vitamin H)*
  Associated with the vitamin B complex, biotin is necessary for the proper utilization of the B vitamins. It is needed for carbohydrate metabolism and for a healthy nervous system. It can help to prevent hair from turning grey and from falling out excessively. It is also useful in relieving skin inflammations and muscle pains.

- *Choline*
  Choline is another member of the vitamin B complex. It helps to control the build-up of cholesterol, and it aids in the transmission of nerve impulses. It also helps to eliminate drugs and poisons through the liver.

- *Inositol*
  Inositol is yet another member of the vitamin B complex. It can help to lower elevated blood cholesterol levels, promote healthy hair and prevent excessive hair loss. It may be useful in combating eczema and in redistributing body fat. It also helps to prevent constipation.

- *PABA (Para-aminobenzoic Acid)*
  This member of the vitamin B complex is important for the health of the blood, skin and intestines. It may prevent wrinkles and has been known to aid in restoring natural colour to the hair. It is also useful in preventing sunburn.

Vitamin C

Vitamin C (like vitamins A and E) is an antioxidant, which helps to slow down the destructive effects of oxygen. It is essential for the formation of collagen, and it is an anti-stress vitamin. It is important for the health of the blood circulation.

Vitamin C is useful in helping to prevent or relieve the symptoms of the common cold, and in reducing the effects of many allergy-producing substances. It facilitates the absorption of dietary iron, and it acts as a natural laxative. In addition, vitamin C helps the body to utilize sugar effectively, and it may be useful in easing uncomfortable menopausal symptoms such as 'hot flushes'.

The best vitamin C sources are fresh fruits such as berries, citrus fruits, kiwi fruit, strawberries and rosehips (the seed pods of wild roses), and fresh vegetables such as cabbage, green and red peppers and mustard and cress.

Associated with vitamin C are a group of substances known as **bioflavonoids**. They occur in the pulp, but not in the juice, of citrus fruits, and particularly in the white of the rind. They facilitate vitamin C absorption and increase its effectiveness. They also help to keep connective tissue healthy and increase the strength of capillary walls. (Capillaries are minute blood vessels.) Other sources of bioflavonoids include apricots, blackberries, buckwheat, cherries and rosehips.

Vitamin D (Calciferol)

Vitamin D regulates the absorption of calcium and phosphorus from the intestines, and aids in the assimilation of vitamin A. Along with vitamins A and C, it can help to prevent colds and it is also useful in relieving eye inflammations.

Vitamin D may be obtained through the action of sunlight on the skin, and from foods such as vitamin D-enriched milk, butter, eggs, fish and fish liver oils.

Vitamin E (Tocopherol)

Vitamin E is a powerful antioxidant and it is also considered an anti-stress nutrient. It is an effective vasodilator (it widens blood vessels and facilitates blood flow). It helps to prevent the formation of blood clots, and it is a natural diuretic.

Vitamin E can help you to look younger by slowing down cellular ageing. It combats fatigue, protects against pollution, and is useful in easing the discomfort of menopausal 'hot flushes'.

Good vitamin E sources include almonds and other nuts, broccoli, Brussels sprouts, eggs, fresh fruits, green leafy vegetables, legumes, seeds, unrefined oils, wheatgerm and whole grains.

EFAs (Essential Fatty Acids)

Two classes of fatty acids are considered essential: omega-3 and omega-6. (Essential in this instance means that the body needs these nutrients but cannot produce them. They therefore have to be provided by the diet.)

EFAs help to prevent a build-up of cholesterol in the arteries; they promote healthy skin and hair; aid in weight reduction by burning saturated fats and they help to prevent prostate gland enlargement.

The best EFA sources are generally the oils of certain seeds and nuts, such as flax (linseed), safflower, sesame, sunflower and evening primrose. Other good sources are corn, peanut and soya bean oils; also almonds, avocados, green leafy vegetables, peanuts, pecan nuts, sunflower seeds, walnuts and whole grains.

Vitamin K (Menadione)

This 'blood vitamin' promotes proper blood clotting and so helps to prevent excessive bleeding. It is also required for the production of the protein matrix upon which calcium is deposited to form bone. (A matrix is the basic substance from which something is made or develops.)

A varied, wholesome diet usually provides enough vitamin K for normal requirements. Rich food sources include alfalfa sprouts, cow's milk, egg yolk, fish liver oils, green leafy vegetables and kelp (a type of seaweed). Other vitamin K sources are sunflower, soya bean and other unrefined vegetable oils.

MINERALS

Boron

Boron helps to safeguard calcium in the body. It appears necessary for activating vitamin D and certain hormones, such as oestrogen. It may be useful in reducing the discomfort of 'hot flushes' and in controlling atherosclerosis.

The safest way to increase your intake of this mineral is to include boron-rich foods in your diet. These include fresh fruits and vegetables such as alfalfa, cabbage, lettuce, peas, snap beans, apples and grapes. Other sources of boron are almonds, dates, hazelnuts, peanuts, prunes, raisins and soya beans.

Calcium

Calcium is an anti-stress mineral needed for the proper functioning of nervous tissue. It is also required for good muscle tone, sound teeth and bones, and for a healthy cardiovascular (heart and blood vessels) system. In addition, calcium helps to metabolize iron and is useful in combating insomnia.

The best food sources of calcium include blackstrap molasses, carob flour (powder), citrus fruits, dried beans, dried figs, green vegetables, milk and milk products, peanuts, sesame seeds, soya beans, sunflower seeds and walnuts.

Chromium
Chromium is needed for proper sugar utilization and may therefore be useful in helping to prevent diabetes. It also aids in lowering elevated blood-pressure.

The best natural sources of chromium include brewer's yeast and corn oil.

Cobalt
Cobalt is part of vitamin B_{12} and is therefore essential for healthy red blood cells.

Good natural sources of cobalt include green leafy vegetables, kelp, torula yeast and whole grains grown in mineral-rich soils.

Copper
Copper helps in the proper functioning of nerve, brain and connective tissue. It is also essential for healthy blood and for the utilization of vitamin C.

If you eat an adequate amount of green leafy vegetables and wholegrain products, you are unlikely to be copper deficient. Other sources of this mineral include legumes, nuts and prunes.

Iodine (Iodide)
Iodine is needed for the health of the thyroid gland, which controls metabolism. It is needed for energy, and may also be useful in weight control. It promotes mental alertness and helps to keep hair, skin and nails healthy.

The best natural iodine sources include broccoli, cabbage, carrots, garlic, lettuce, onions, pineapple, and foods grown in iodine-rich coastal soils.

Iron
Iron is necessary for the proper metabolism of the B vitamins and for the assimilation of vitamin C. It is required for healthy blood and for a sound immune system.

Good iron sources include blackstrap molasses, brewer's yeast, Brussels sprouts, cauliflower, dried fruits, egg yolk, kiwi fruit, leafy vegetables, seaweed, seeds, Sharon fruit (persimmon), strawberries, watermelon, wheatgerm and whole grains.

Caution Avoid taking an iron supplement unless it has been prescribed by a doctor: excess iron can accumulate in the body and interfere with immunity.

Magnesium
Magnesium is an anti-stress mineral that is useful in combating depression. It is essential for protein synthesis and for the utilization of several nutrients. Magnesium is also needed for sound bones, for a healthy nervous system and for the health of the heart and blood vessels.

The best magnesium sources include fresh fruits and vegetables grown in mineral-rich soils, almonds and other nuts eaten fresh from the shell, seeds and whole grains and cereals.

Manganese
Manganese is necessary for the body's proper use of biotin, vitamin B_1 and vitamin C. It is needed for sound bones and for the production of thyroxine, the principal hormone of the thyroid gland. Manganese is also important for the proper digestion and utilization of food and for the health of the nervous system.

The best natural manganese sources include beets, egg yolks, green leafy vegetables, nuts, peas and wholegrain cereals.

Molybdenum
This mineral forms a vital part of the enzyme responsible for the body's iron utilization. It also promotes general well-being.

The best food sources of molybdenum include dark-green leafy vegetables, legumes and whole grains.

Phosphorus
Phosphorus is needed for the health of the nervous system and also for sound bones and teeth.

Good food sources include corn, low-fat dairy products, dried fruits, egg yolk, legumes, nuts, seeds and whole grains.

Potassium

Potassium works with the mineral sodium to regulate the body's water balance and to normalize heart rhythms. It is needed for muscles and nerves to function properly. Potassium can also contribute to clarity of thinking by improving the oxygen supply to the brain. In addition, this mineral helps to dispose of body wastes and is useful in lowering high blood-pressure.

The best sources of potassium are foods in their natural state. These include bananas, citrus fruits, aubergine (eggplant), mint leaves, nuts, pears, peas, peppers, watercress, watermelon and wholegrain cereals.

Selenium

Selenium is an antioxidant that is also required for healthy blood circulation. It helps to preserve the youthful elasticity of the body's tissues, and it can relieve 'hot flushes' and other menopausal discomforts.

Selenium requirements are greater for men than for women: almost half of men's selenium supply is concentrated in the testes and parts of the seminal ducts.

The best food sources of this mineral include apple cider vinegar, asparagus, brewer's yeast, eggs, garlic, mushrooms, sesame seeds, unrefined cereals, wheatgerm, whole grains and whole-grain products.

Silicon (Silica)

This anti-ageing nutrient gives life to the skin, lustre to the hair and beautiful finishing touches to the whole body. It is needed for healthy bones and connective tissue. It is also required for the normal functioning of the adrenal glands (involved in stress reactions) and for the health of the heart and blood vessels.

Foods made from natural buckwheat are a rich source of silicon, but the mineral may also be obtained from a variety of fresh fruits and vegetables and from wholegrains and cereals.

Sodium

Sodium is necessary for normal heart function and, along with potassium and the mineral chlorine, for keeping body fluids near a natural pH (in chemistry, the degrees of acidity or alkalinity of a substance are expressed in pH values).

Natural sodium sources include asparagus, beets, carrots, celery, courgettes (zucchini), raw egg yolk, figs, marrow (squash), oatmeal, string beans and turnips.

Sulphur

Sulphur helps to maintain the oxygen balance necessary for proper brain function. It is also essential for healthy hair, skin and nails, and for the synthesis of collagen.

Food sources include beans, bran, Brussels sprouts, cabbage, egg yolk, garlic, horseradish, kale, onions, peppers of all kinds, and radishes.

Vanadium

Vanadium is thought to be involved in the storage of excess calories in the form of fat, and even a marginal deficiency may result in weight gain.

Vanadium is also involved in sugar utilization, and may in addition inhibit cholesterol build-up.

This mineral is found primarily in plant foods such as radishes, and in other unrefined foods.

Zinc

Zinc is essential for the proper functioning of more than seventy enzyme systems. It is important for a healthy immune system and for mental and physical health in general.

Zinc helps muscles to contract normally; it helps in the formation of insulin; it has a normalizing effect on prostate gland function; it promotes mental alertness, and it keeps skin, nails and blood circulation healthy.

Foods rich in zinc include brewer's yeast, cheese, eggs, green and lima beans, mushrooms, non-fat dried milk, nuts, pumpkin seeds, soya beans, sunflower seeds, wheatgerm and wholegrain products.

OTHER NUTRIENTS

Carnitine

Carnitine is an amino acid (protein building-block), the main function of which is to transport fatty acids into the 'powerhouses' of tissue cells to generate energy.

Carnitine is needed for the health of the heart and blood vessels, for mental alertness and for better tolerance of exercise.

There are two forms of carnitine: D-carnitine, which is biologically inactive and L-carnitine, which is active and which is obtainable mostly from animal foods. Some carnitine, however, is provided by dairy products, avocado and tempeh.

Note Should you decide to take a carnitine supplement, use *only* L-carnitine.

Lecithin

Lecithin improves fat metabolism. It breaks down fats and cholesterol in the blood so that they may be utilized effectively by the body's cells.

The best lecithin sources include unrefined foods containing oil, such as nuts, soya beans and wheat. Eggs also contain lecithin: the lecithin content of a fertile egg is about 1700 milligrams.

EATING FOR LONG LIFE

As the years go by, you are likely to experience significant changes in your living situation, such as children leaving home, loss of income, moving or the loss of a spouse. Such changes may affect what and how you eat. For example, living in unfamiliar surroundings or not having anyone with whom to share a meal can result in dietary neglect or, on the other hand, in overeating to compensate for sadness or loneliness.

It is important to remember that continuing to eat a variety of foods, in reasonable amounts, promotes and preserves health, keeps weight normal and contributes to the joy of living. A well-nourished body recovers better from illness than one that is malnourished and debilitated.

Remember also that taking mineral and vitamin supplements indiscriminately is not the answer to good health and long life. Check with your dietitian, doctor or other qualified therapist.

Here are tips to help you to stay fit for many years:

- Eat a good breakfast to give you energy for the day.
- Reduce your intake of high-fat foods, which have been associated with serious health disorders, such as heart and blood vessel diseases.
- Avoid high-protein diets. They impose extra demands on the body and may compromise your immune system. They cause increased excretion of important nutrients such as calcium, and create a greater than usual need for others, such as the B vitamins.
- Give preference to low-fat milk products which provide calcium and high-quality protein, but which are lower in fat and calories than whole-milk products.
- Eat plenty of complex carbohydrates such as fresh fruits and vegetables, potatoes and wholegrain breads and pasta to provide bulk and important nutrients, to keep bowel function regular and to promote and preserve a trim, healthy body.
- Have a meal of beans or lentils once or twice a week. These are high-fibre, low-fat foods that provide inexpensive yet good-quality protein.
- Avoid using over-processed foods, such as many convenience foods which lack essential nutrients. Read labels. Avoid foods with added sugar, salt and fat.

- Reduce the salt (sodium) you add to food during preparation, cooking and at the table. A high-sodium intake has been linked to hypertension (high blood-pressure).
- Reduce your consumption of refined sugars, which have been implicated in conditions such as high cholesterol, diabetes, obesity and tooth decay.
- Decrease caffeine intake or even eliminate it altogether. Instead, drink water, unsweetened fruit juices, freshly-pressed vegetable juices, herbal teas and low-fat milk.
- Avoid substances known to be antagonistic to essential nutrients, for example, commercial laxatives, alcohol and tobacco.
- If you experience symptoms of hypoglycaemia (low blood sugar), eat five or six small meals, evenly spaced throughout the day, rather than three larger meals, to help to maintain adequate blood sugar levels.
- Shop for foods with high nutrient content. Store, prepare and cook them so as to conserve their nutrients (consult any good book on nutrition or cooking).
- Occasionally pack a picnic lunch and invite a friend to share it with you in a nearby park. The fresh air will do wonders for your appetite and spirits, and so will companionship.
- Be good to yourself: lay the table with care. Add a vase of fresh flowers when possible, or a lighted candle. Put on some pleasing music to create an atmosphere that is conducive to good appetite and feelings of well-being. Ask a friend to dine with you.
- Take your time. Relax for a short while before your meal. Eat slowly and savour your food. Avoid overeating.

8

HELP FOR COMMON DISORDERS

Certain changes and health problems are inevitable as the human body ages. But the ageing process can be influenced by making use of the powerful mind-body connection. Biological age (i.e. how old your body is in terms of cellular processes) is changeable: regular physical exercise, for example, can reverse several of the most typical effects of biological ageing, including hypertension (high blood-pressure), excess body fat, faulty sugar metabolism and decreased muscle mass. In fact, gerontologists (specialists in the study of ageing) have found that older adults who adopt healthy lifestyle habits improve the quality of their life and also their life expectancy by about ten years.

There are ten markers for age which are reversible:

1 *Aerobic capacity.* (Aerobic exercise is that in which the energy needed is supplied by the oxygen breathed in. Aerobic exercise is required for sustained periods of hard work and vigorous athletic activity.)
2 *Basal metabolic rate.* Basal metabolism is the amount of energy needed to maintain life when you are at digestive, physical and emotional rest.
3 *Body fat.*
4 *Body temperature regulation.*

5 *Bone density.*
6 *Blood-pressure.*
7 *Blood sugar* (glucose) *tolerance.* This refers to your ability to metabolize glucose.
8 *Cholesterol/HDL ratio.*
9 *Lean body* (muscle) *mass.*
10 *Strength.*

A few very simple lifestyle changes can help you to keep looking and feeling young. These include:

• Taking steps to promote sound, refreshing sleep at night.
• Eating adequate amounts of wholesome foods, rich in essential nutrients (eating breakfast is important).
• Maintaining weight that is normal for you (and no more than 10 per cent above that if you are a woman, or 20 per cent above that if you are a man).
• Exercising regularly, including outdoor exercise such as walking.
• Not smoking and not drinking alcohol (or drinking only moderately).

By regularly incorporating into your activities of daily living the various techniques offered in this book, and by applying the nutritional suggestions, you can acquire significant control over the way you age.

Remarkable advances in modern medical knowledge, practice and technology, combined with the body's innate power of self-healing, have given us the potential to transform our later years into a time of excellent health, vitality and self-fulfilment.

COMMON DISORDERS

This chapter describes symptoms of common disorders often associated with the years beyond fifty. For various other disorders, and exercises and nutrients to help in their management, please refer to my book entitled *Yoga Therapy* (*see* the bibliography for details).

Symptoms are perceptible changes in the body or in its functions, which may indicate disease or a phase of disease. After each entry, references are given to exercises that can help to prevent the disorder from arising or worsening, or aid in a return to normal function. Each exercise is followed by a figure number, which refers to the illustration of the posture (exercise). The postures have been arranged alphabetically for your convenience, and are to be found in Chapters 3 and 4.

It is important to warm up before and cool down after practising the postures (*see* Chapter 3). A review of Chapter 2 is also suggested, to be clear as to how best to prepare for the exercises and what cautions to observe. All the breathing techniques are described in Chapter 5, and the 'mental' exercises such as meditation are presented in Chapter 6.

Also listed after each entry are nutrients that are particularly beneficial for the specific condition. Some of their chief food sources are given in Chapter 7. Please remember that all nutrients work together. Please also consult a dietitian, nutritionist or other qualified professional before you decide to take nutritional supplements.

The nutrients, exercises and other techniques suggested in this chapter will help to strengthen and mobilize your body's natural self-healing resources, to help to prevent or reverse disease and to assist in a return to and maintenance of normal function. The suggestions are in no way a substitute for competent medical care. It is imperative that you *consult a doctor* trained in orthodox medicine if you have a serious health problem, whether it is acute or longstanding. Combining the best that orthodox medicine has to offer, with yoga techniques and good nutrition, will greatly enhance your chances of a long and healthy life.

ANXIETY

Anxiety, which is a feeling of apprehension, dread, worry or uneasiness, is a normal reaction to a perceived threat to one's body, loved ones, values or way of life. Often, the cause is not easy to identify.

A certain amount of anxiety is considered normal, as it can stimulate an individual to act purposefully. Excessive anxiety, on the other hand, impedes normal functioning.

Symptoms of anxiety, which can sometimes be frightening, include difficulty in breathing, pain over the heart, palpitations, tightness of the throat and other forms of muscle tension, headaches and pressure in the head, hand tremors, feeling cold, agitation and feelings of being out of control, sweating, nausea, diarrhoea, generalized weakness and feeling faint, and inability to think clearly or to concentrate.

If breathing becomes too rapid, it can lead to hyperventilation (overbreathing) and thence to alkalosis, in which body fluids become excessively alkaline.

Exercises
The Cobra (Fig. 10), Forwards Bend, Sitting (Fig. 18), The Plough (Fig. 31), Pose of Tranquillity (Fig. 32), Spinal Twist (Fig. 34), Sun Salutations (Figs. 36–44). Also: Alternate Nostril Breathing (Fig. 52), Anti-Anxiety Breath, Cleansing Breath, Humming Breath, Sighing Breath.

Nutrients

The B vitamins, especially B_1, B_3, B_6, biotin and PABA; calcium and magnesium.

ARTHRITIS

Arthritis is the inflammation of joints. It is often accompanied by pain and swelling, and frequently also by a change in the structure of the joints. It affects the hands, spine, hips, feet and other weight-bearing joints.

Arthritis may result from, or be associated with, conditions which include infection, rheumatic fever, ulcerative colitis, disorders of the nervous system, degenerative joint diseases, metabolic disturbances such as gout, neoplasms (new growths), inflammation of structures near the joints (such as bursitis), and various other conditions, including psoriasis and Raynaud's disease.

Exercises

Exercise is vital to success in managing arthritis, and yoga is ideal. If you do not exercise, your pain will increase as your muscles weaken and your joints stiffen.

Warm-ups, including The Butterfly (Fig. 1), Lying Twist (Fig. 2) and The Flower (Fig. 3); The Bow (Fig. 7), Chest Expander (Fig. 9), The Cobra (Fig. 10), The Eagle (Fig. 16), Forwards Bend, Sitting (Fig. 18), Forwards Bend, Standing (Fig. 19), Half Moon (Fig. 20), The Plough (Fig. 31), Pose of Tranquillity (Fig. 32), Spinal Twist (Fig. 34), Squatting Posture (Fig. 35), Sun Salutations (Figs. 36–44), Toe-Finger Postures (Figs. 45, 46, 47), Triangle Posture (Fig. 50). Also: Alternate Nostril Breathing (Fig. 52), Anti-Anxiety Breath, Bellows Breath, Cleansing Breath, Complete Breath. Meditation.

Nutrients

Vitamin A, the B vitamins, especially B_1, B_2, B_5, B_6 and B_{12}, vitamin C and bioflavonoids, vitamins D and E, EFAs, boron, calcium, copper, iron, magnesium, manganese, selenium, silicon and zinc.

Note Avoid foods and drinks known to interfere with the absorption of minerals, such as bran, coffee and tea.

Some arthritis sufferers find relief from their symptoms when they eliminate from their diet foods from the nightshade family, namely, aubergine (eggplant), peppers, potatoes and tomatoes. (Tobacco also belongs to this family.)

ATHEROSCLEROSIS

Atherosclerosis refers to an abnormal thickening of arteries due to a build-up of fats in their inner walls. (Arteries are vessels that carry blood from the heart to the tissues.) Although the causes of this condition are not entirely known, factors that play a part include hypertension, high cholesterol levels, cigarette smoking, diabetes and obesity.

Physical and emotional stress can accelerate atherosclerosis. Regular exercise is a splendid way to improve circulation, counteract stress and reduce the risk of atherosclerosis. Giving up smoking is also advisable.

Dietary measures to combat atherosclerosis include avoiding refined foods, saturated fats and alcohol, and increasing the intake of complex carbohydrates. Also suggested is the liberal use of garlic and onions, which have protective properties.

Exercises

The Fountain (Fig. 5), Chest Expander (Fig. 9), Corrective Prayer Posture (Fig. 11), The Fish (Fig. 17), Half Moon (Fig. 20), The Mountain (Fig. 29), Pose of Tranquillity (Fig. 32), The Shoulderstand (Fig. 33), Spinal Twist (Fig. 34), Sun Salutations (Figs. 36–44), Holy Fig Tree Posture (Fig. 49). Also: Alternate Nostril Breathing (Fig. 52), Anti-Anxiety Breath, Cleansing Breath, Humming Breath, Sighing Breath. Meditation.

Nutrients

The B vitamins, especially B_3, B_6, B_9, B_{15}, choline and inositol, vitamin C and bioflavonoids, vitamin E, EFAs, boron, calcium, chromium, copper, magnesium, selenium, silicon, vanadium, zinc, fibre, lecithin and carnitine.

BACKACHE

Backache may occur in any of the areas on either side of the spine, from the neck to the pelvis. It is usually characterized by a dull, continuous pain and by muscle tenderness. The pain sometimes radiates to the legs.

The causes of backache are numerous and include infection, tumours, disorders of the spine, fractures, strains or sprains, muscle injury, spasm or inflammation, poor postural habits and emotional factors.

Please refer to my book entitled *The Yoga Back Book* (see the bibliography) for detailed information on back care.

Exercises

When not in pain, regularly practise: Lying Twist (Fig. 2), Rock-and-Roll (Fig. 4), Fountain (Fig. 5), The Bow (Fig. 7), The Bridge (Fig. 8), The Cobra (Fig. 10), Corrective Prayer Posture (Fig. 11), Curling Leaf (Fig. 13), Dancer's Pose (Fig. 14), Dog Stretch (Fig. 15), Forwards Bend, Sitting (Fig. 18), Half Moon (Fig. 20), Inclined Plane (Fig. 22), Knee Press (Fig. 24), The Locust (Fig. 25), The Mountain (Fig. 29), Pelvic Stretch (Fig. 30), The Plough (Fig. 31), Pose of Tranquillity (Fig. 32), Spinal Twist (Fig. 34), Squatting Posture (Fig. 35), Toe-Finger Postures (Figs. 45, 46, 47), Triangle Posture (Fig. 50), Yoga Sit-Up (Fig. 51). Also: Alternate Nostril Breathing (Fig. 52), Anti-Anxiety Breath, Breathing Away Pain (for pain relief), Cleansing Breath, Complete Breath, Humming Breath, Sighing Breath. Meditation.

Nutrients

Vitamin A, the B vitamins, Vitamins C, D and E, boron, calcium, fluorine, magnesium, phosphorus and silicon.

CONSTIPATION

Difficulty or infrequency of bowel elimination is known as constipation. But how often defaecation should occur varies greatly, and in healthy adults it may range from two to three bowel movements a day to two per week.

Factors contributing to constipation include failure to establish regular times for bowel movements; anxiety, worry or fear; a sedentary lifestyle; inadequate fluid intake; a low-fibre diet; excessive use of laxatives; drugs that are constipating; poor abdominal musculature; tumours and other intestinal lesions (local diseased parts).

Note A change in bowel habits should be discussed with a doctor.

Exercises

Lying Twist (Fig. 2), Rock-and-Roll (Fig. 4), The Fountain (Fig. 5), The Bow (Fig. 7), The Cobra (Fig. 10), Curling Leaf (Fig. 13), The Fish (Fig. 17), Forwards Bend, Sitting (Fig. 18), Half Moon (Fig. 20), Half Shoulderstand (Fig. 21), Inclined Plane (Fig. 22), Knee Press (Fig. 24), The Locust (Fig. 25), The Mountain (Fig. 29), Pelvic Stretch (Fig. 30), The Plough (Fig. 31), Pose of Tranquillity (Fig. 32), The Shoulderstand (Fig. 33), Spinal Twist (Fig. 34), Squatting Posture (Fig. 35), Sun Salutations (Figs. 36–44), Toe-Finger Postures (Figs. 45, 46, 47), Triangle Posture (Fig. 50), Yoga Sit-Up (Fig. 51). Also: Alternate Nostril Breathing (Fig. 52), Anti-Anxiety Breath, Bellows Breath, Complete Breath. Candle Concentration (Fig. 53).

Nutrients

The B vitamins, especially B_1, B_5, B_9, choline, inositol and PABA, vitamin C, magnesium, potassium, fibre and plenty of water.

DEPRESSION

The criteria for diagnosing depression include the presence of at least four of the following symptoms, occurring every day for at least two weeks: poor appetite; significant weight loss or gain; insomnia or sleeping too much; low energy levels and fatigue; loss of interest or pleasure in one's usual activities; decreased sex drive; feelings of worthlessness; self-reproach or inappropriate guilt feelings; poor concentration; feelings of hopelessness, and suicidal thoughts.

Exercises

Graduate exercises according to your energy level. Start with warm-ups. Add one or two sets of Sun Salutations (Figs. 36–44), done slowly, as your energy increases. Practise the Pose of Tranquillity (Fig. 32) daily.

When you feel ready, add the Alternate Leg Stretch (Fig. 6), The Bridge (Fig. 8), Chest Expander (Fig. 9), Corrective Prayer Posture (Fig. 11), Curling Leaf (Fig. 13), Half Moon (Fig. 20), Half Shoulderstand (Fig. 21), Knee Press (Fig. 24), The Mountain (Fig. 29), Pelvic Stretch (Fig. 30), The Shoulderstand (Fig. 33), Spinal Twist (Fig. 34), Squatting Posture (Fig 35), Toe-Finger Posture, Lying (Fig. 45), The Tree (Fig. 48), Holy Fig Tree Posture (Fig. 49) and the Yoga Sit-Up (Fig. 51).

Daily practice of any of the following is also suggested: Alternate Nostril Breathing (Fig. 52), Anti-Anxiety Breath, Cleansing Breath, Complete Breath. Candle Concentration (Fig. 53).

Nutrients

The B vitamins, especially B_1, B_2, B_3, B_5, B_6, B_9, B_{12}, biotin, choline, inositol and PABA, vitamin C, calcium, iron, magnesium, potassium and zinc.

Note If you suspect that low blood sugar (which is a common cause of depression) may be contributing to a persisting low mood, consider eating five or six small nutritious meals, spaced evenly throughout the day, instead of three larger meals. *Check with your doctor.*

DIABETES MELLITUS

Diabetes mellitus (commonly known as diabetes) is a disorder of carbohydrate metabolism, and is characterized by high blood sugar and glucose (sugar) in the urine.

Although the basic cause of diabetes is still unknown, the direct cause is failure of beta cells of the pancreas to secrete an adequate amount of insulin. In most instances, diabetes is the result of a genetic disorder, but it may also be due to a deficiency of beta cells caused by inflammation, malignancy or surgery.

Common in middle life is adult-onset diabetes, in which insulin is produced but not properly utilized. Fortunately, most diabetics in this category can control the disorder by a combination of weight loss (if they are overweight), a diet that provides all the essential nutrients and which is high in fibre and complex carbohydrates, regular exercise and effective stress management.

To decrease the risk of complications from diabetes, the following measures are suggested:

- Stop smoking.
- Have regular medical check-ups (controlling hypertension is important).
- Have regular dental check-ups. Keep your teeth and gums healthy.
- Take measures to keep your eyes healthy. Have them checked about once a year. Report changes in vision.
- Take care of your feet: wash them regularly and dry them well, especially between the toes (make sure that the water temperature is not hot, so as to prevent burns). Apply moisturizing cream to dry skin.

  Do not cut calluses and corns yourself. Consult a foot doctor. Also report cuts that do not heal. Wear shoes that fit well, and always check for the presence of foreign objects in them. Do not walk with bare feet. Wear cotton or woollen socks and change them daily. *Do not use* hot-water bottles.

Exercises

Exercising one hour after meals can help to lower blood glucose levels. Exercise should be planned to suit your own physical capability, and is most beneficial when done at about the same time and for the same length of time each day.

Regular exercise increases blood circulation to all parts of the body and may decrease the chances of cardiovascular disease, such as that which leads to heart attacks and strokes. Exercise may also aid in curbing the appetite and so contribute to a gradual weight loss. In addition, regular exercise can help to relieve stress, which affects blood glucose levels. *Consult with your doctor* about an exercise programme that is appropriate for you.

The following yoga exercises are generally useful: The Fountain (Fig. 5), The Bow (Fig. 7), The Cobra (Fig. 10), Corrective Prayer Posture (Fig. 11), Curling Leaf (Fig. 13), The Fish (Fig. 17), Forwards Bend, Sitting and Standing (Figs. 18, 19), Half Moon (Fig. 20), Half Shoulderstand (Fig. 21), The Plough (Fig. 31), Pose of Tranquillity (Fig. 32), The Shoulderstand (Fig. 33), Spinal Twist (Fig. 34), Sun Salutations (Figs. 36–44), Holy Fig Tree Posture (Fig. 49). Also: Alternate Nostril Breathing (Fig. 52), Bellows Breath, Humming Breath, Sighing Breath. Meditation.

Nutrients

Vitamin A, the B vitamins, especially B_1, B_2, B_3, B_5, B_6, B_{12} and inositol, vitamin C and bioflavonoids, vitamin E, EFAs, chromium, copper, iodine, magnesium, manganese, phosphorus, potassium, selenium, vanadium, zinc, carnitine and fibre.

Note Taking any supplement that can affect blood sugar regulation is potentially dangerous, especially for diabetics who need to take insulin. *Always check with your doctor.*

EYE PROBLEMS

Dry-eye syndrome is thought to be a form of collagen disease and is common among post-menopausal women. The chief symptoms include rheumatoid arthritis, dry mouth and dry eyes. Other symptoms associated with this disorder are increased dental caries, dryness of the vagina, excessive loss of scalp hair, and disturbances of the heart, lungs, kidneys, nervous and digestive systems. The dominant feature of these conditions is tissue dehydration, and so an adequate daily fluid intake is essential.

Eyestrain is tiredness of the eyes because of over-use. Causes include stress, pollution and spending a great deal of time before computer screens. Eyestrain can lead to other problems, such as eye inflammations and headaches.

Diligent eye care can help to keep eyestrain to a minimum, thus limiting the potential for permanent damage. If problems already exist, yoga practice can help to slow down the rate of deterioration of the eyesight and bring about improvement of existing disorders.

Relaxation is a key to improving eye function. Eye muscles, like muscles elsewhere in the body, respond to stress by over-contracting. This can impair focusing, distort the shape of the eyeball and worsen other vision problems. General relaxation combined with eye exercises can help to reduce tension and strain, and build up the stamina of the eye muscles.

Macular degeneration is another eye problem. The macula is the central part of the retina of the eye. It is responsible for fine vision. Degeneration of the macula is a leading cause of decreased visual acuity.

Although the cause of this condition is not entirely known, heredity and the normal process of ageing are contributing factors. Risk factors for the development of macular degeneration include cigarette smoking, poor nutrition, atherosclerosis and hypertension.

Exercises

Neck and shoulder warm-ups. Curling Leaf (Fig. 13), Half Shoulderstand (Fig. 21), Pose of Tranquillity (Fig. 32), The Shoulderstand (Fig. 33), Spinal Twist (Fig. 34), Sun Salutations (Figs. 36–44). Also: Alternate Nostril Breathing (Fig. 52), Cleansing Breath, Complete Breath, Sighing Breath. Candle Concentration (Fig. 53).

Additional Exercises
Palming

Palming helps to counteract eyestrain and prevent a build-up of tension in your face and body. It also promotes concentration and may be useful in combating insomnia.

1 Sit naturally erect at a desk, table or anywhere that allows you to rest your elbows comfortably.

2 Rub your palms together vigorously, to warm them and charge them with natural electricity.

3 Rest your palms gently over closed eyes. *Do not* put pressure on your eyeballs. Breathe regularly.

4 Stay in this position for a minute or two to begin with; longer as you become more practised.

5 Separate your fingers to re-introduce the light slowly. Relax your arms and hands.

To finish the exercise, blink several times if you wish, to lubricate the eyes with natural fluid.

The Clock

1 Sit tall. Keep your head, shoulders and hands still. Breathe regularly throughout the exercise.

2 Imagine looking at a large clock in front of you. Look at twelve for about one second; look at each subsequent number for one second, going in a clockwise direction. Look straight ahead. Rest.

3 Repeat step 2, proceeding in an anti-clockwise direction this time.

The Clock helps to strengthen your eye muscles and keep them healthy. It also helps to relieve eyestrain.

Focusing Exercises

1 Look at a distant object, such as a tree top or church spire.

2 Slowly shift your gaze to a nearby object.

3 Repeat steps 1 and 2, several times in smooth succession, remembering to breathe regularly throughout the exercises.

Note Look for opportunities throughout the day to practise the above eye exercises. Take breaks from reading and other close work, or from watching television or sitting before a computer screen. Also practise the exercises outdoors whenever you can, to benefit in addition from the fresh air.

Nutrients
Vitamin A, the B vitamins especially B_2 and inositol, vitamins C, D and E, EFAs, selenium and zinc.

FATIGUE

Feelings of weariness, weakness or exhaustion may occur as a result of various conditions which include excessive activity, malnutrition, circulatory problems, respiratory disorders, endocrine gland disturbances, infectious diseases, emotional upsets, physical disability or environmental noise.

Exercises
Your exercise programme should be designed so as to build up your energy gradually. Start with warm-ups and short daily walks. As your energy increases, add one or two sets of Sun Salutations (Figs. 36–44), done slowly. Each day, practise some of the following (always include the Pose of Tranquillity): Chest Expander (Fig. 9), Corrective Prayer Posture (Fig. 11), Curling Leaf (Fig. 13), Half Moon (Fig. 20), Half Shoulderstand (Fig. 21), The Mountain (Fig. 29), Pose of Tranquillity (Fig. 32), the Shoulderstand (Fig. 33), Spinal Twist (Fig. 34), Holy Fig Tree Posture (Fig. 49). Also: Alternate Nostril Breathing (Fig. 52), Anti-Anxiety Breath, Bellows Breath, Breathing Away Fatigue (a modification of Breathing Away Pain), Cleansing Breath, Humming Breath, Sighing Breath. Candle Concentration (Fig. 53). Meditation.

Nutrients
Vitamin A, the B vitamins, especially B_1, B_5, B_6, B_9, B_{12}, B_{15}, biotin and PABA, vitamins C and E, EFAs, calcium, cobalt, copper, iodine, iron, magnesium, manganese, molybdenum, potassium, phosphorus, selenium, silicon and zinc.

FLATULENCE

Excessive gas in the stomach and intestines is known as flatulence. It may produce belching, bloating and abdominal pain.

In older adults, intestinal gas (wind) is likely to be due to a deficiency of enzymes necessary for digesting carbohydrates in milk, fruits or vegetables. Dental defects, such as missing teeth or poorly-fitting dentures, cause air to be swallowed and food to be chewed improperly. Gas may also be a symptom of lactose intolerance (intolerance of milk).

Some vegetables, such as aubergine (eggplant), Brussels sprouts, cabbage, cauliflower, onions and turnips are often referred to as 'strong-flavoured'. They are frequently thought to be responsible for producing flatulence and therefore avoided. This is unfortunate because they are rich in nutrients.

Problems should not arise when these and similar vegetables are eaten raw or stored, prepared and cooked properly.

Experiments have shown that when these vegetables are cooked for eight to ten minutes, not above boiling, almost no sulphur compounds break down which can form gases during digestion to cause discomfort. If the chilled vegetables are diced or shredded, they can be thoroughly cooked within ten minutes. When longer cooking is required, such as when cauliflower is cooked whole, the vegetable should be simmered in milk to neutralize plant acids, and so prevent the breakdown of sulphur compounds.

In short, when plant acids are not leached out through soaking; when cooking temperatures are kept low and cooking time kept to a minimum, the so-called strong-flavoured vegetables are surprisingly mild-flavoured and sweet.

Exercises
Rock-and-Roll (Fig. 4), The Bow (Fig. 7), The Cobra (Fig. 10), Curling Leaf (Fig. 13), Knee Press (Fig. 24), The Locust (Fig. 25), Pose of Tranquillity (Fig. 32), Squatting Posture (Fig. 35), Yoga Sit-Up (Fig. 51). Perineal Exercise (*see* Urinary Problems, page 78). Also: Alternate Nostril Breath (Fig. 52), Anti-Anxiety Breath, Bellows Breath, Breathing Away Pain (for pain relief), Complete Breath.

Nutrients
The B vitamins, especially B_1, B_3, B_5, vitamin K and potassium.

Note *Avoid* the following, which introduce air and gas into your body: chewing gum, drinking carbonated beverages, drinking from water fountains and smoking.

HAIR LOSS
It is normal to lose between twenty and sixty hairs daily. When hair loss becomes excessive, however, it is known as *alopecia*. It is linked to a number of conditions, including heredity, ageing, illnesses, infectious diseases, hormonal imbalance, nervous system disorders, toxic substances (including some drugs), dandruff, impaired blood circulation, poor nutrition and stress.

Exercises
Rock-and-Roll (Fig. 4), The Bow (Fig. 7), Forwards Bend, Standing (Fig. 19), Half Shoulderstand (Fig. 21), Pose of Tranquillity (Fig. 32), The Shoulderstand (Fig. 33), Spinal Twist (Fig. 34). Also: Alternate Nostril Breathing (Fig. 52), Anti-Anxiety Breath, Bellows Breath, Complete Breath, Sighing Breath. Meditation.

Nutrients
Vitamin A, the B vitamins, especially B_5, B_9, biotin, inositol and PABA, EFAs, calcium, cobalt, copper, magnesium, selenium, silicon, sulphur and zinc.

HYPERTENSION (HIGH BLOOD-PRESSURE)
Blood-pressure refers to the force that blood exerts against the inner walls of arteries as a result of the heart's pumping action. Hypertension is a condition in which the blood-pressure is higher than that judged to be normal.

Because hypertension generally produces no symptoms, many people are unaware that they have the condition until they have a routine medical examination. However, untreated hypertension can lead to serious illness, such as coronary artery disease, stroke and other cardiovascular (heart and blood vessels) disorders.

For many years yoga breathing, relaxation and meditation techniques have been used successfully as an adjunct to other treatments to help to lower blood-pressure and to keep it within normal range. Outstanding among the techniques in this respect is the Pose of Tranquillity.

Exercises
Pose of Tranquillity (Fig. 32), Palming (*see* the entry on Eye Problems), Alternate Nostril Breathing (Fig. 52), Anti-Anxiety Breath, Cleansing Breath, Complete Breath, Humming Breath, Sighing Breath. Candle Concentration (Fig. 53), and all the meditative exercises.

Nutrients
Vitamin A, the B vitamins, especially B_2, B_3, B_6, B_{15}, choline and inositol, vitamin C and bioflavonoids, vitamin E, EFAs, calcium, chromium, magnesium, potassium, silicon, vanadium, zinc and lecithin.

Note *Avoid* cigarette smoking and alcohol. Limit salt, fat and caffeine intake. Increase your intake of potassium-rich foods (such as aubergine, pears, peas and peppers). Use garlic liberally: it provides vitamins A and C and several minerals; it helps to reduce cholesterol build-up; it gives diameter to blood vessels, and it is useful in lowering high blood-pressure.

INSOMNIA
Insomnia is the inability to sleep. It also refers to sleep that ends prematurely, or which is interrupted by periods of wakefulness.

As we grow older, sleep patterns tend to change and we generally need less sleep than we did when we were younger.

Although insomnia is not a disease, it may be a symptom of disease and should be investigated. Some causes are anxiety, depression and pain.

Exercises
The Cobra (Fig. 10), Forwards Bend, Sitting (Fig. 18), The Mountain (Fig. 29), Pose of Tranquillity (Fig. 32), Spinal Twist (Fig. 34), Sun Salutations (Figs. 36–44). Also: Alternate Nostril Breathing (Fig. 52), Anti-Anxiety Breath, Breathing Away Pain (for pain relief), Cleansing Breath, Complete Breath, Humming Breath, Sighing Breath. Candle Concentration (Fig. 53). Meditation.

Nutrients
The B vitamins, especially B_1, B_3, B_5, B_6, biotin, choline and inositol, calcium, magnesium and potassium.

Note *Avoid* beverages containing caffeine. Try a glass of warm milk (it contains calcium and also tryptophan, an amino acid that helps to induce sleep).

Check any medications you are prescribed: some can contribute to insomnia.

MENOPAUSAL PROBLEMS
Menopause is the period that marks the permanent cessation of menstrual activity. It usually occurs between the ages of 35 and 58 years.

Symptoms associated with menopause include hot flushes (or flashes), excessive perspiration, chills, nervousness, mood swings, depression, low energy, fatigue, heart palpitations, dizziness and headaches. Many of these symptoms are thought to be linked to a decline in the production of the hormone oestrogen.

Exercises
The Butterfly (Fig. 1), Lying Twist (Fig. 2), Rock-and-Roll (Fig. 4), The Fountain (Fig. 5), The Bow (Fig. 7), Chest Expander (Fig. 9), The Cobra (Fig. 10), Cross Beam (Fig. 12), The Fish (Fig. 17), Forwards Bend, Sitting (Fig. 18), Knee and Thigh Stretch (Fig. 23), The Mountain (Fig. 29), Pelvic Stretch (Fig. 30), The Plough (Fig. 31), Pose of Tranquillity (Fig. 32), Spinal Twist (Fig. 34),

Squatting Posture (Fig. 35), Sun Salutations (Figs. 36–44), Holy Fig Tree Posture (Fig. 49), Yoga Sit-Up (Fig. 51). Also: Alternate Nostril Breathing (Fig. 52), Anti-Anxiety Breath, Bellows Breath, Cleansing Breath, Complete Breath, Sighing Breath. Perineal Exercise (*see* Urinary Problems, page 78).

Nutrients
Vitamin A, the B vitamins, especially B_5 and B_6, vitamin C and bioflavonoids, vitamins D and E, boron, EFAs, calcium, chromium, iodine, iron, magnesium, selenium, silicon and zinc.

OSTEOPOROSIS
Osteoporosis is a bone-loss disorder that affects mainly post-menopausal women and, to a lesser degree, sedentary men. The condition is marked by decreased bone density as bone breaks down faster than it is being formed.

Bone loss occurs in all parts of the skeleton, with the greatest loss taking place in spongy rather than in compact bone. Particularly serious are bone losses in the spine and femur (upper leg bone). The vertebrae (bones of the spine) may become compressed and vulnerable to fractures.

Although the exact cause of decreased bone mass in older adults is unknown, associated factors include heredity, the amount of bone mass present at skeletal maturity, exercise, nutrition and diminished oestrogen production.

Exercises
The following postures, combined with regular walking and other forms of weight-bearing exercise such as dancing, are useful in helping to prevent osteoporosis or to slow down its progression: Lying Twist (Fig. 2), Dancer's Pose (Fig. 14), The Eagle (Fig. 16), Forwards Bend, Standing (Fig. 19), Half Moon (Fig. 20), Half Shoulderstand (Fig. 21), The Shoulderstand (Fig. 33), Spinal Twist (Fig. 34), Squatting Posture (Fig. 35), Sun Salutations (Figs. 36–44), Toe-Finger Posture, Standing (Fig. 47), The Tree (Fig. 48), Holy Fig Tree Posture (Fig. 49), Triangle Posture (Fig. 50). Alternate Nostril Breathing (Fig. 52).

Nutrients
Vitamin A, vitamin B_9, vitamin C and bioflavonoids, vitamins D and K, boron, calcium, copper, fluorine, magnesium, manganese, phosphorus, silicon and zinc.

Notes *Avoid* high-protein diets as they leach minerals, including calcium, from the body. Eliminate from your diet refined sugar, caffeine and alcohol. Stop smoking, as it is associated with accelerated bone loss. Cigarettes also lower oestrogen levels in women, thus increasing the risk of osteoporosis. Smokers have been found to be doubly at risk of hip fractures than non-smokers.

Also *avoid* foods high in oxalic acid (so-called 'calcium blotters'), such as almonds, beetroot tops, cashew nuts, peanuts, rhubarb and spinach. (Oxalic acid inhibits calcium absorption.)

PAIN
Pain is a protective mechanism for our bodies. It can be acute as in an injury, or chronic as in arthritic conditions. Pain-relieving medications, which are called *analgesics*, sometimes produce undesirable side effects and some are habit-forming.

Some people seem to cope better with pain than others, and the 'spinal gate control theory' may offer an explanation for this. Simply explained, there appears to be a nervous mechanism that in effect opens or closes a 'gate' that controls pain stimuli travelling to the brain for interpretation. This mechanism can be influenced by certain psychological factors including attitude, anxiety, tension, power of suggestion and personality.

Natural pain control methods, such as yoga practices, are largely based on closing the spinal 'gate' so that pain stimuli do not reach the brain. When compared with pain management using drugs, these natural methods are safer: they work by mobilizing the body's own resources to promote comfort and a sense of well-being, and they are free of unwanted side effects.

A close relationship exists between our respiratory (breathing) system and our perception of and reaction to pain. Breathing speeds up and becomes shallow when we are uncomfortable or in pain, and it may even become irregular or difficult. When we are at ease, however, it tends to be slower and regular.

Yoga techniques train you in the conscious, voluntary control of your breathing, so that you can slow it down at will to relieve tension and anxiety, thereby decreasing fear and pain. In addition, they provide a mental distraction from the pain itself, so that it is perceived as less intense.

Exercises

Regular exercise makes available more of the body's natural pain relievers (endorphins and enkephalins). The following yoga practices are useful in the effective management of pain and discomfort:

Corrective Prayer Posture (Fig. 11), Dancer's Pose (Fig. 14), The Eagle (Fig. 16), Toe-Finger Posture, Standing (Fig. 47), The Tree (Fig. 48), Holy Fig Tree Posture (Fig. 49). Alternate Nostril Breathing (52) and Candle Concentration (Fig. 53), which train you in mental steadiness.

The Pose of Tranquillity (Fig. 32), practised daily, will discourage a build-up of tension and teach you to relax completely from head to toes.

All the breathing exercises, especially Breathing Away Pain, are suitable for pain control. Daily meditation is also recommended.

Nutrients

Vitamin A, the B vitamins, especially B_1, B_3, B_6, B_9, B_{12} and biotin, vitamins C and E, calcium, copper, magnesium and selenium.

PROSTATE GLAND PROBLEMS

The prostate gland encircles the neck of the urinary bladder and urethra in males. It secretes a thin, opalescent, slightly alkaline fluid that is a component of semen.

Prostate gland enlargement is common, particularly after middle age. This produces bothersome symptoms such as frequent urination (often at night), inability to empty the bladder completely and difficulty or pain when passing urine.

Cancer of the prostate gland is also common, especially after 50 years of age. In the early stages there are no symptoms. Later, however, symptoms mimic those of prostate gland enlargement, as the growing tumour restricts the flow of urine. Blood may also appear in the urine.

Exercises

To help to keep your prostate gland healthy, practise as many as possible of the following every day or every other day:

The Butterfly (Fig. 1), Lying Twist (Fig. 2), Rock-and-Roll (Fig. 4), The Fountain (Fig. 5), Half Shoulderstand (Fig. 21), Knee and Thigh Stretch (Fig. 23), Knee Press (Fig. 24), The Locust (Fig. 25), Pelvic Stretch (Fig. 30), The Shoulderstand (Fig. 33), Spinal Twist (Fig. 34), Squatting Posture (Fig. 35), Sun Salutations (Figs. 36–44), Toe-Finger Posture, Lying (Fig. 45), Holy Fig Tree Posture (Fig. 49). Also: Alternate Nostril Breathing (Fig. 52), Anti-Anxiety Breath, Breathing Away Pain (for pain relief), Cleansing Breath, Complete Breath, Sighing Breath. Meditation.

Nutrients

Vitamins A, C and E, EFAs, selenium, zinc and fibre.

Note *Avoid* drinks containing caffeine. Caffeine is diuretic and so increases urinary discharge. Also reduce your intake of alcohol and fats.

Sitz Baths

Sitz baths are useful in relieving congestion associated with prostate gland enlargement. Here is one way to prepare a sitz bath:

- Fill a large, deep basin with enough water to cover your pelvic area when you sit in it.
- Keep the water temperature between 38°C and 46°C (100°F and 115°F).
- Keep your legs out of the water. Keep your upper body warm to prevent chilling.
- Stay in the sitz bath for ten to twenty minutes. Repeat the bath one or more times during the course of a day.

SKIN PROBLEMS

Some skin problems respond well to simple treatments and minor changes in diet. Others require medication and therapies best given or recommended by a doctor or specialist (dermatologist).

Exercises

The Fountain (Fig. 5), Corrective Prayer Posture (Fig. 11), Curling Leaf (Fig. 13), Dog Stretech (Fig. 15), Forwards Bend, Standing (Fig. 19), Half Moon (Fig. 20), Half Shoulderstand (Fig. 21), The Mountain (Fig. 29), Pose of Tranquillity (Fig. 32), The Shoulderstand (Fig. 33), Spinal Twist (Fig. 34), Sun Salutations (Figs. 36–44), Holy Fig Tree Posture (Fig. 49). Also: Alternate Nostril Breathing (Fig. 52), Anti-Anxiety Breath, Bellows Breath, Complete Breath, Sighing Breath. Meditation.

Nutrients

Vitamin A, the B vitamins, especially B_2, B_3, B_6, biotin, inositol and PABA, vitamins C, D and E, EFAs, chromium, copper, magnesium, selenium, silicon, sulphur, zinc and fibre. It is important to drink plenty of water.

URINARY PROBLEMS

The urinary system includes the kidneys, ureters, bladder and urethra, i.e. structures that are responsible for the secretion and elimination of urine.

Increased urinary frequency may be due to nervous excitement, inflammation of the bladder, disease of the spinal cord or enlarged prostate gland.

Decreased urination occurs after sweating, diarrhoea and bleeding, and may also be a result of brain disease, drug poisoning and inflammation of the kidneys.

Incontinence refers to the inability to fully control the flow of urine. It is more common in older than in younger adults. In stress incontinence, urine escapes when you cough, sneeze, laugh, jog or stand up suddenly. Some medications can contribute to urinary incontinence. *Check with your doctor.*

Exercises

Avoid strenuous exercise, but practise as many of the following as you comfortably can every day or every other day:

The Butterfly (Fig. 1), Lying Twist (Fig. 2), The Bow (Fig. 7), The Bridge (Fig. 8), The Cobra (Fig. 10), The Locust (Fig. 25), Pelvic Stretch (Fig. 30), Pose of Tranquillity (Fig. 32), Spinal Twist (Fig. 34), Squatting Posture (Fig. 35). Also: Alternate Nostril Breathing (Fig. 52), Anti-Anxiety Breath, Breathing Away Pain (for pain relief), Cleansing Breath, Complete Breath, Sighing Breath.

Perineal exercise

The so-called Kegel exercises (often recommended for pregnant women) are based on the age-old yoga perineal exercise which follows. Practised every day, it will help to improve the tone of your pelvic musculature.

1 Sit, lie or stand comfortably. Breathe regularly.
2 *Exhale* and tighten your perineum (the area between your anus and your external genitals), as if to prevent a bowel movement or the passage of urine.
3 Hold the tightening as long as your exhalation lasts.
4 Inhale and relax, breathing regularly.
5 Repeat steps 2 to 4 once. Repeat it later.

Note Practise the Perineal Exercise several times throughout the day. Practise it anywhere that you feel comfortable doing it: when travelling by bus, car, train or aeroplane; while waiting at traffic lights; in a queue; at boring parties and meetings. No one will know what you are doing.

Nutrients
Vitamin A, the B vitamins, especially B_2, B_5, B_6, B_9, B_{12}, choline and PABA, vitamin C and bioflavonoids, vitamins D and E, EFAs, calcium, magnesium, selenium and zinc.

Drink plenty of water unless you suffer from urinary incontinence. If you do, limit your intake to about four glasses a day, unless you have some other medical condition that requires otherwise. Eliminate drinks containing caffeine.

Also avoid irritants such as spicy foods and carbonated beverages. Include cranberry juice; it has been found beneficial in some bladder conditions, because of its acid content.

Note A number of substances can irritate the bladder and should therefore be avoided when possible. These include perfumes in soaps, bubble baths, toilet paper and feminine hygiene products.

Empty your bladder regularly. A full bladder is more liable to leak than one that is not full, and it is also more vulnerable to infection.

GLOSSARY

Acid-base balance The mechanisms by which the acidity and alkalinity of body fluids are kept in a state of equilibrium.

Adrenal glands Two small triangular-shaped endocrine glands, one above each kidney.

Amino acids Building-blocks of proteins and neurotransmitters ('chemical messengers').

Anaemia Deficiency in either the quality or quantity of circulating red blood cells.

Analgesic A remedy that relieves pain.

Angina pectoris Severe pain and constriction that occurs suddenly in the region of the heart, due to insufficient blood supply to the coronary arteries. The pain usually radiates to the left shoulder and down the left arm.

Antioxidant An agent that prevents or inhibits oxidation.

Arteriosclerosis A gradual loss of elasticity in the walls of arteries, due to thickening and calcification.

Artery One of the vessels carrying blood from the heart to the tissues.

Asana A posture comfortably held; a yoga physical exercise.

Biological age How old your body is in terms of cellular processes, and vital signs such as blood-pressure.

Capillary A minute blood vessel connecting an artery and a vein.

Carcinogen An agent that incites or produces cancer.

Cardiovascular Pertains to the heart and blood vessels.

Cartilage Gristle. A specialized type of connective tissue forming parts of the skeleton, and covering the ends of bones.

Catalyst A substance that speeds up the rate of a chemical reaction without itself being permanently altered in the reaction.

Cholesterol A sterol (fat) widely distributed in animal tissues, oils and other foods. Also found in various parts of the human body.

Chronological age How old you are according to the calendar, i.e. in years.

Collagen A fibrous insoluble protein found in connective tissue, including skin. It represents about 30 per cent of total body protein.

Connective tissue Tissue that supports and connects other tissues and body parts.

Coronary Refers to the heart.

Defaecation Evacuation of the bowels.

Discs Refers to spinal discs, which cushion the bones making up the spine (vertebrae).

Diuretic An agent that increases the secretion of urine.

Electrolytes Ionized salts in blood, tissue fluids and cells including salts of sodium, potassium and chlorine.

Endocrine glands Glands whose secretions (hormones) flow directly into the blood and are circulated to all parts of the body.

Enzymes Complex proteins that are capable of inducing chemical changes in other substances without being changed themselves.

Free radicals Highly reactive oxygen atoms, 'mischievous molecules' that damage cells. They are considered a first step in cancer development.

Gastrointestinal Pertains to the stomach and intestine.

Haemoglobin The iron-containing pigment of red blood cells.

Haemorrhage Abnormal internal or external discharge of blood.

Hamstring muscles ('hamstrings') Three muscles at the back of the thighs. They flex the legs, and extend the thighs and draw them towards the mid-line of the body.

HDL High-density Lipoprotein. 'Good cholesterol'.

Hormone A chemical substance which is generated in one organ and carried by the blood to another, in which it excites activity. A secretion of endocrine glands.

Hypertension High blood-pressure.

Immune system The body's chief specific defence against disease and other foreign agents. It includes white blood cells, bone marrow, the lymphatic system, the spleen and the thymus gland.

Inorganic Occurring in nature, independent of living things. Also indicates chemical compounds that do not contain carbon.

Insulin The endocrine secretion of the pancreas, which regulates sugar metabolism and ensures complete fat combustion.

Kelp A member of the seaweed family. An excellent source of iodine and other minerals, and also vitamins A, C, D and several B vitamins.

Laxative A food or chemical that facilitates the elimination of bowel contents, and thereby counteracts constipation.

Legumes Fruits or pods of beans, peas or lentils.

Lesion An injury, wound or diseased area of the body.

Lymph The fluid from the blood which has passed through the walls of capillaries to supply nutrients to tissue cells.

Macula The small part of the eye's retina, where the highest number of light-sensing cells are concentrated. Disease in this area, called macular degeneration, is a leading cause of blindness.

Metabolism The sum of all the chemical changes that take place within an organism.

Metabolite Any product of metabolism.

Mucous membranes Membranes lining passages and cavities connected directly or indirectly with the skin.

Neurological Refers to the nervous system.

Neurotransmitter A chemical messenger which conveys electrical impulses from one nerve cell (neuron) to another.

Oestrogen An endocrine secretion which stimulates the female generative organs to reproductive function.

Oral Pertains to the mouth.

Organic Refers to an organ or organs. Pertaining to or derived from animal or vegetable forms of life. Also denotes chemical substances containing carbon.

Osteomalacia A disease characterized by painful softening of bones. (Osteomalacia is the adult form of rickets, which is due particularly to a deficiency of vitamin D.)

Oxidation The process of a substance combining with oxygen.

Oxygenation Saturation or combination with oxygen, as the aeration of the blood in the lungs.

Pancreas A gland which lies behind the stomach. It secretes a digestive fluid (pancreatic juice) which acts on all classes of foods, and it also secretes the hormone insulin.

Parasympathetic nervous system Part of the autonomic nervous system. It consists of certain fibres and some cranial nerves (originating in the brain). Some effects of parasympathetic stimulation are constriction of the pupil of the eye and slowing of the heart rate.

pH Potential of Hydrogen. In chemistry, the degrees of acidity or alkalinity of a substance are expressed in pH values. A neutral substance has the pH of 7.

Physiology The science of the functions of living bodies.

Prana Vital breath. Vitality.

Pranayama Refers to the integration of the nervous and respiratory (breathing) systems. Breathing exercises.

Precursor A parent substance from which another substance is made chemically. A forerunner.

Respiratory Pertains to respiration, or breathing.

Retina The innermost coat of the eyeball, which receives images formed by the lens (of the eye), and is the immediate instrument of vision.

Serotonin A chemical thought to be involved in neural (nerve) mechanisms which are important in sleep and sensory perception.

Sympathetic nervous system A large part of the autonomic nervous system. Stimulation of the sympathetic nervous system produces reactions such as the constriction of blood vessels in the parts supplied, a general rise in blood-pressure and acceleration of heartbeat. In general, these activities are associated with a response to fright, fight or flight.

Synthesis In chemistry, the union of elements to produce compounds; the process of building up.

Thyroid gland A two-lobed endocrine gland situated in front of the windpipe (trachea).

Toxin A poisonous substance of plant or animal origin.

Uptake The absorption of a nutrient, chemicals and medicines by tissues or by an entire organism.

Vasodilator Causing relaxation of the blood vessels. A nerve or drug that dilates (widens) the blood vessels.

BIBLIOGRAPHY

A'nanda Ma'rga. *Teaching Asanas*. Los Altos Hills, California: Amrit Publications, 1973.

Anderson, Kenneth. *Symptoms After 40*. New York: Arbor House, 1987.

Ballentine, Rudolf, M., Jr, M.D. (Ed.). *Joints and Glands Exercises* (as taught by Sri Swami of the Himalayas). Honesdale, Pennsylvania: The Himalayan International Institute of Yoga Science and Philosophy, 1977.

B.C. Ministry of Health and Ministry Responsible for Seniors. *Reach for Health*, 1988.

Carper, Jean. *Stop Aging Now!* New York: HarperCollins, 1995.

Chopra, Deepak, M.D. *Boundless Energy*. New York: Harmony Books, 1995.

— *Ageless Body, Timeless Mind*. New York: Harmony Books, 1993.

Cooper, Kenneth, MD. 'Antioxidants: 20th Century Medicine.' Burnaby, Canada: *Alive Canadian Journal of Health and Nutrition*, No. 158, December 1995, pp. 13–15.

Davis, Adelle. *Let's Stay Healthy. A Guide to Lifelong Nutrition*. San Diego, California: Harcourt Brace Jovanovich, 1983.

— *Let's Eat Right to Keep Fit*. London: Thorsons, 1970.

— *Let's Cook It Right*. New York: The New American Library, 1970.

Devereux, Godfrey. *The Elements of Yoga*. Shaftesbury, Dorset: Element Books, 1994.

DeVries, Herbert A., Ph.D., with Hales, Dianne. *Fitness After 50*. New York: Charles Scribner's Sons, 1982.

Ebersole, Priscilla, Ph.D., RN, FAAN, and Hess, Patricia, Ph.D., RN-C, GNP. *Toward Healthy Aging* (4th ed.). (Human Needs and Nursing Response.) St. Louis: Mosby, 1990.

Eichenlaub, John E., MD. *Prime Time. A Doctor's Guide to Staying Younger Longer*. Englewood Cliffs, New Jersey: Prentice Hall, 1993.

Eliopoulos, Charlotte. *Gerontological Nursing*. (3rd ed.). Philadelphia: J.B. Lippincott, 1993.

Feinstein, Alice (Ed.). *Training the Body to Cure Itself*. Emmaus, Pennsylvania: Rodale Press, 1993.

Fromm, Erich. *The Art of Loving*. New York: Bantam, 1963.

Giller, Robert M., and Matthews, Kathy. *Natural Prescriptions*. New York: Ballantine Books, 1994.

Gordon, James S., MD. 'Holistic Medicine.' *The Encyclopedia of Healing*. New York: Chelsea House, 1988.

Hawranik, Pamela, RN, MN, Ph.D.(e), and Walker, Jan, RN, BN. 'Targeting Seniors'. Ottawa, Canada: *The Canadian Nurse*, August 1995, pp. 35–39.

Heckheimer, Estelle F., RN, MA. *Health Promotion of the Elderly in the Community*. Philadelphia: W.B. Saunders, 1989.

Hoffer, Abram, MD, Ph.D., and Walker, Morton, DPM. *Nutrients to Age Without Senility*. New Canaan, Connecticut: Keats Publishing, 1980.

Kaufmann, Klaus. *Silica: The Forgotten Nutrient*. Burnaby, B.C., Canada: Alive Books, 1990.

Lobay, Douglas, ND. *21st Century Natural Medicine*. Kelowna, Canada: Apple Communications, 1992.

Mindell, Earl. *Earl Mindell's Vitamin Bible*. New York: Warner Books, 1979.

Ornish, Dean, M.D. *Dr. Dean Ornish's Program for Reversing Heart Disease*. New York: Random House, 1990.

Parsons, Steve. 'The Power of Breathing.' Burnaby, B.C., Canada: *Alive Canadian Journal of Health and Nutrition*, No. 161, March 1996, pp. 32–33.

Passwater, Richard A. *Super-Nutrition*. New York: Pocket Books, 1975.

Peterson, Vicki. *The Natural Food Catalog*. New York: Arco Publishing, 1978.

Province. 'New Age of Yoga.' Vancouver, Canada: *Province Showcase*, October 31, 1994, pp. B6 and B7.

Purna, Dr Svami. *Balanced Yoga*. Shaftesbury, Dorset: Element Books, 1992.

Roe, Daphne, A. *Geriatric Nutrition* (3rd ed.). Englewood Cliffs, New Jersey: Prentice Hall, 1983.

Rossman, Isadore, MD, Ph.D. *Looking Forward: The Complete Medical Guide to Successful Aging*. New York: E. P. Dutton, 1989.

Tzu, Lao. *Tao Teh Ching* (translated by John C.H. Wu). Boston: Shambhala, 1989.

Wade, Carlson. *Eat Away Illness*. New York: Parker Publishing, 1992.

Weller, Stella, *Yoga Therapy*. London: Thorsons, 1995.

— *The Yoga Back Book*. London: Thorsons, 1993.

— *Santé Immunitaire Naturelle*. Geneva: Éditions Jouvence, 1991.

— *Cuidado Natural del Cabello, Piel y Uñas*. Madrid: Edaf, 1989.

Winter, Ruth, M.S. *A Consumer's Guide to Medicines in Food*. New York: Crown Trade Paperbacks, 1995.

INDEX

Of further interest...

Principles of Yoga

Cheryl Isaacson

Yoga is a time-honoured system of balancing mind, body and spirit. Originally part of the mystical wisdom of Indian philosophy, Western cultures have mostly emphasized its physical practices. These are, however, only one aspect of the integrated way of life which yoga provides. This introduction explains:

- how yoga postures fit into the total yoga system
- ways to use yoga thought and action in daily life
- simple methods for relaxing and meditating
- how to take charge of your own health and energy
- the secrets of personal peace and stability

Yoga for Children

Stella Weller

Yoga for Children is a practical workbook offering stretching and strengthening yoga exercises for children which:

- encourage an awareness of what is happening inside and outside the body
- develop attentiveness and concentration
- build self-esteem and self-confidence
- promote harmony between body and mind
- create a well-adjusted child

Ideal for maintaining firm muscles and flexible joints and for encouraging good posture, these exercises provide even the shyest and least athletically-inclined children with the opportunity to express their feelings and give free rein to their imagination through body movement.

With illustrations and posture names to which children can relate, *Yoga for Children* is comprehensive, easy-to-follow and not only invaluable for parents of 5–15 year olds but also an excellent resource for teachers and other educators.

Yoga Therapy

Safe, natural methods to promote healing and restore health and well-being

Stella Weller

Yoga Therapy offers a safe, effective approach to mobilizing your own built-in healing resources to complement the care provided by your doctor or other therapist.

With the help of clear illustrations you'll learn techniques to help create favourable conditions for the body's own inner forces to bring about remission or healing. These include:

- safe, simple, controlled stretching exercises done with concentration and synchronized breathing to help you develop alertness to early warning signs of illness
- exercises to help you stop smoking, prevent major back problems, overcome menopausal difficulties, lose weight, combat fatigue, cope with anxiety, insomnia, depression, etc
- numerous breathing and relaxation techniques you can incorporate into daily schedules to help you cope effectively with stress

Also included is nutrition information, such as important nutrients and their food sources, to give nutritional support to the healing process and maintain good health.

Yoga for Women

Paddy O'Brien

Yoga for Women is about the advantages and resources yoga has to offer women both as a system of exercise and as an opportunity for self-development and exploration. It is a book for today's woman, whether trying to balance the challenges of family or the demands of work with her own inner needs.

Yoga needs no special equipment, it is not competitive and will help you set aside time for yourself. It will enable you to cope with the stresses of life and explore conflicts about self-image and self-esteem in a gentle, untraumatic way. By enhancing your flexibility, strength and power, it will also give you access to inner peace and tranquillity. It is valuable when feeling fragile, physically vulnerable or undermined, and enriches times of confidence, exuberance and celebration.

The book includes:

- a system of exercises to celebrate womanhood
- a basic yoga 'vocabulary' of postures and breathing
- a programme of postures for life passages from adolescence through pregnancy to old age

It is suitable for complete beginners as well as those with experience and is clearly illustrated with photographs and line drawings.

Shiatsu for Women
The complete guide to restoring health, vitality and well-being

Ray Ridolfi and Susanne Franzen

Giving and receiving relaxing and therapeutic touch is the essence of this increasingly popular healing art. The basics are easy to learn and the simple techniques often give profound results. You'll feel stress just melt away!

Originating from traditional Japanese medicine, shiatsu literally means 'finger pressure'. Pressure and stretching techniques are applied along the body's energy channels, encouraging self-healing, rebalancing the body, and easing both mental and physical tension.

Suitable for the complete beginner as well as those with experience, this book is an excellent practical guide to shiatsu, with an emphasis on women's health concerns. Including both basic self-treatment and shiatsu for two, it will show you how shiatsu can help with:

- pregnancy and childbirth
- menstrual and gynaecological problems
- beauty and sexuality
- common complaints, such as backache and headache

Principles of Shiatsu

Chris Jarmey

Shiatsu is an Eastern therapeutic technique which uses pressure to enhance the flow of life energy – or ki – within the body. This introductory guide is ideal for the beginner or student of this increasingly popular therapy, and for anyone with a serious interest in bodywork. In this accessible and informative book, experienced shiatsu practitioner Chris Jarmey explains the concept of ki, the power which unifies and animates the channels as they are used in shiatsu, the basic treatment techniques and how shiatsu can help specific ailments.

I See Myself in Perfect Health
Your essential guide to self-healing

David Lawson

This is an easy to use book that will benefit anyone who wishes to transform their life. David Lawson, the acclaimed healer and workshop leader, has created a completely new guide to self-healing, filled with exercises, ideas and practical suggestions that really work.

Including:
- the way to become your own healer and counsellor
- how to tap the powers of your mind for health and joy
- finding the courage to take charge of your own personal happiness
- using the power of self-healing to improve your health

PRINCIPLES OF YOGA	0 7225 3212 1	£5.99	☐
YOGA FOR CHILDREN	0 7225 32067	£7.99	☐
YOGA THERAPY	0 7225 2998 8	£9.99	☐
YOGA FOR WOMEN	1 85538 426 4	£8.99	☐
SHIATSU FOR WOMEN	1 85538 482 5	£9.99	☐
PRINCIPLES OF SHIATSU	0 7225 3362 4	£5.99	☐
I SEE MYSELF IN PERFECT HEALTH	1 85538 485 x	£7.99	☐

All these books are available from your local bookseller or can be ordered direct from the publishers.

To order direct just tick the titles you want and fill in the form below:

Name: _____

Address: _____

_____

_____

Postcode:_____

Send to: Thorsons Mail Order, Dept 3, HarperCollins*Publishers*, Westerhill Road, Bishopbriggs, Glasgow G64 2QT.
Please enclose a cheque or postal order or your authority to debit your Visa/Access account –

Credit card no: _____

Expiry date: _____

Signature: _____

– to the value of the cover price plus:
UK & BFPO: Add £1.00 for the first book and 25p for each additional book ordered.
Overseas orders including Eire: Please add £2.95 service charge. Books will be sent by surface mail but quotes for airmail despatches will be given on request.

24 HOUR TELEPHONE ORDERING SERVICE FOR ACCESS/VISA CARDHOLDERS –
TEL: 0141 772 2281.